Essential Oils & Aromatherapy

WORKBOOK

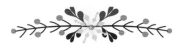

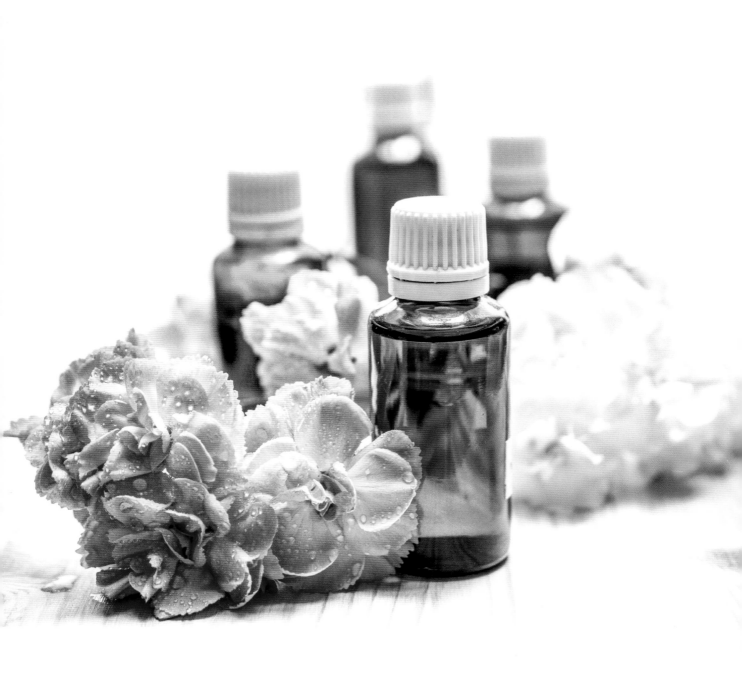

Essential Oils &
Aromatherapy
WORKBOOK

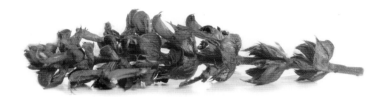

MARCEL LAVABRE

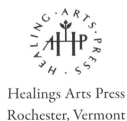

Healings Arts Press
Rochester, Vermont

Healing Arts Press
One Park Street
Rochester, Vermont 05767
www.HealingArtsPress.com

Healing Arts Press is a division of Inner Traditions International

Originally published in 1990 by Healing Arts Press under the title *Aromatherapy Workbook*
Revised and expanded second edition published in 1996 by Healing Arts Press

Note to the reader: *This book is intended as an informational guide. The remedies, approaches, and techniques described herein are meant to supplement, and not to be a substitute for, professional medical care or treatment. They should not be used to treat a serious ailment without prior consultation with a qualified health care professional.*

Cataloging-in-Publication Data for this title is available from the Library of Congress

ISBN 978-1-64411-070-6 (print)
ISBN 978-1-64411-071-3 (ebook)

Printed and bound in India by Replika Press Pvt. Ltd.

10 9 8 7 6 5 4 3 2 1

Text design and layout by Virginia Scott Bowman
This book was typeset in Garamond Premier Pro with Argent, Helvetica, and Gill Sans used as display typefaces

To send correspondence to the author of this book, mail a first-class letter to the author c/o Inner Traditions • Bear & Company, One Park Street, Rochester, VT 05767, and we will forward the communication.

✦ ✦ ✦

To my daughter, Melissa

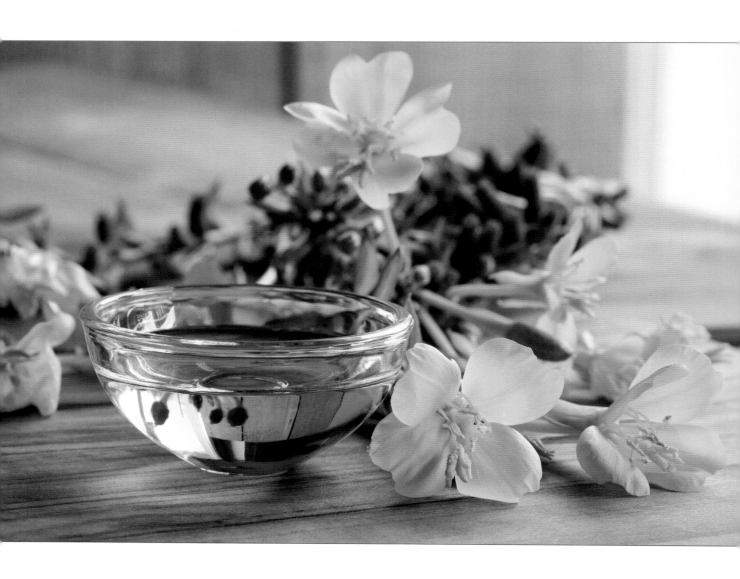

Contents

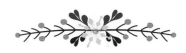

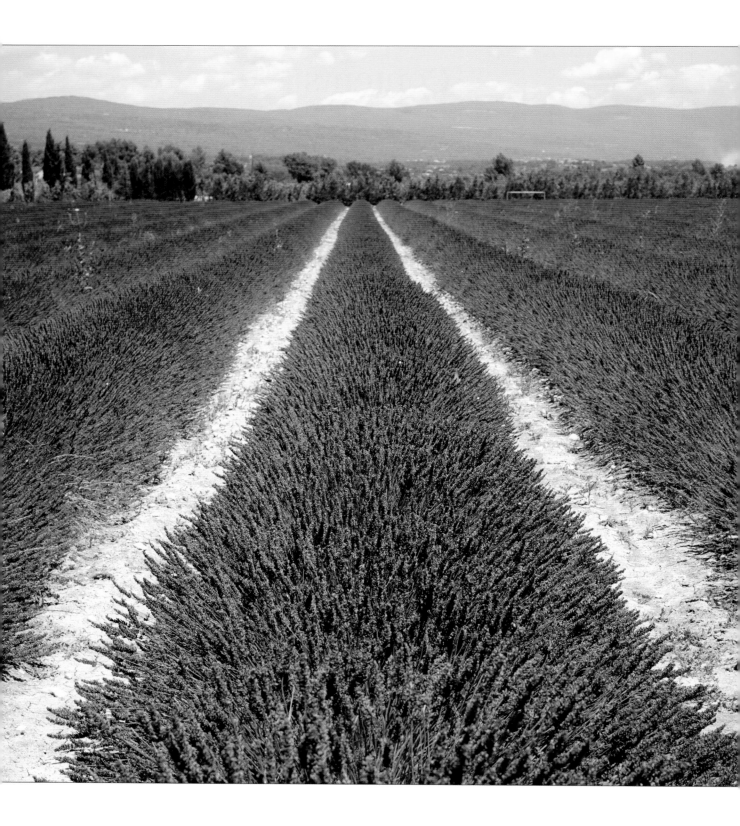

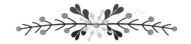

From "Aroma-What" to Buzzword

The Evolution of Aromatherapy

Born in 1950, I grew up on a small farm in the Quercy region of southern France at a time when the French countryside was about to undergo a radical transformation. My father was still plowing the earth with oxen when I was born, but he had bought his first tractor by the time I was three years old. We practiced subsistence farming, with a real menagerie of domestic animals, producing most of the food we needed for our own consumption, growing a little bit of everything, from the cash crops of wheat, oats, barley, and corn to all types of fruits and vegetables. We even had a small vineyard and a tiny plot of lavender.

Harvests, the highlights of the year, were a feast for the senses, starting with hay at the end of spring, followed by cherries, wheat, oats, and barley all the way to grapes, corn, apples, and walnuts in autumn, but the lavender harvest was always my favorite. The whole family would gather in the field and start cutting as soon as the morning dew had dried. We loaded the lavender onto a trailer, and we kids would all jump on top of the heap and ride to the distillery, bathing all the way in the sweet, fresh, herbal-floral fragrance.

The distillery is where the magic happened. The lavender was loaded into huge vats (at least they looked huge to us little kids), and big furnaces sent steam up through the lavender. The steam collected in the *col de cygne* (swan-necked lid) and passed down through the *serpentin* (condenser coil), and by the time it was all said and done, the big heap of lavender had been transformed into a flask of golden-green liquid with a characteristically sweet fragrance. But if anybody had asked me back then about "aromatherapy," I most likely would have responded with an incredulous "Aroma-what?"—or rather, "Aroma-*quoi*?"

Our family doctor at the time prescribed more tisanes (herbal teas) and vitamins than antibiotics and painkillers, but if you had asked him about "alternative medicine," he most likely

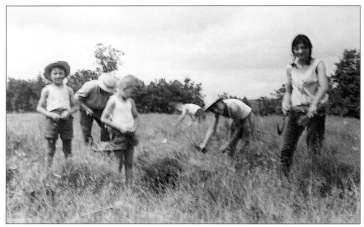

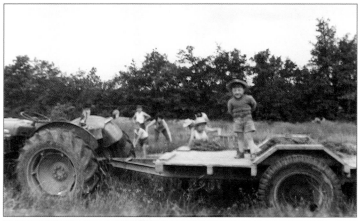

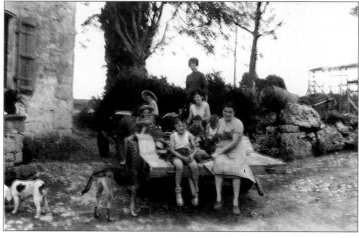

*Marcel Lavabre (as a child) and family harvesting lavender on
the family farm in southern France circa 1960*

would have replied, "Alternative to what?"

Meanwhile, the French chemist and scholar René-Maurice Gattefossé had discovered the healing power of the essential oil of lavender when he famously burned himself in his laboratory in 1910. He coined the term *aromatherapy* and published his seminal book on the subject in 1937.

Jean Valnet was a French military surgeon posted to Tonkin from 1950 to 1953 during the Indochina War (which segued into the Vietnam War when the United States joined in and tried to outdo the French, with the same lack of success). The French army in Indochina often lacked even basic supplies, such as medicines and weaponry, and Valnet began experimenting with local essential oils and other aromatic and herbal preparations to treat the most severe wounds in his patients, with well above average results. His founding work, *Aromathérapie: Traitement des maladies par les essences des plantes,* first published in 1964 and later published in English as *The Practice of Aromatherapy,* is still one of the primary references on the subject.

I became familiar with aromatherapy in the mid-1970s, when I moved to the Jabron Valley, near Sisteron in the Provence region of southeastern France. The farmers there who had been collecting medicinal plants and distilling essential oils for hundreds of years had a deep knowledge of their virtues. Every mother and grandmother had her special recipes to cure all types of ailments, and they were eager to share their knowledge as the new generations were leaving this beautiful but impoverished region for the lure of the big cities.

Staffed by my horse and a mischievous donkey, I started a small enterprise harvesting wild medicinal herbs and distilling all kinds of plant material. I liked experimenting. One of my neighbors was Henri Viaud, an eccentric and fascinating gentleman-farmer, distiller, and publisher, among other occupations, with a past worthy of a cloak-and-dagger novel. Another neighbor was Pierre Lieutaghi, a living botanical encyclopedia. From Henri, Pierre, and many others, I learned a lot about herbs and their power. I should mention Madam Garcin, an outspoken healer with a witch's tendencies, who held the secret to heal burns and snakebites as well as an encyclopedic knowledge of folk medicine. Together with her son Gilles, I crisscrossed the Luberon valley and the adjoining Montagne de Lure (Lure Mountain) in search of linden, wild lavender, hyssop, thyme, savory, oregano, mugwort, wormwood, and all the bountiful aromatic and medicinal plants abounding in that region.

I moved to Boulder, Colorado, in 1981, with a suitcase full of essential oils of my own production and a few diffusers. I was intent on starting a new aromatherapy venture in the United States, but when I approached prospective customers I was met with an incredulous "Aroma-what?" punctuated by blank stares. It took me three months to make my first sale to an adventurous chiropractor who bought a diffuser and few essential oils for his waiting room.

I soon realized that education was the key

and started giving lectures and seminars, first in front of sparse audiences, then in classrooms that began to fill up with eager students. I gave lectures and seminars all over the United States and all over the world, especially in Japan, Hong Kong, Singapore, Korea, and Indonesia. In Latin America, I gave seminars in Mexico, Buenos Aires, and even Campinas, near São Paulo, Brazil.

I moved to Los Angeles in 1987 and joined forces with fellow aromatherapists and aromatherapy entrepreneurs to create the American AromaTherapy Association (AATA). I was charged with organizing the third AATA convention on April 29 and 30, 1990, with my then marketing director and future partner in teaching, my good friend Michael Scholes. Featuring the who's who of aromatherapy at the time—with speakers like Dr. Jean-Claude Lapraz and Dr. Daniel Pénoël, both from France; Patricia Davis, Jan Kusmirek, Robert Tisserand, and Valerie Worwood, all from the United Kingdom; Yugal Luthra and Prakash Purohit of India; and Victoria Edwards, Avery Gilbert, Mindy Green, Kurt Schnaubelt, Michael Scholes, and myself from the USA—the convention was a resounding success. Attendees came from all over the world, from Norway to New Zealand, Japan, China, and South Africa. The convention intended to build bridges and marked a turning point in the evolution of aromatherapy in the United States.

Times have changed since the "Aromawhat?" and the blank stares!

A quick Google search of the word

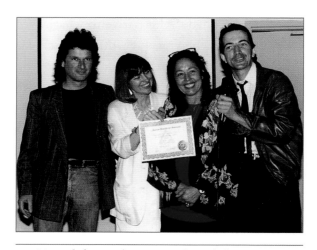

From left to right: Kurt Schnaubelt, Victoria Edwards, Jeanne Rose, and Marcel Lavabre. Kurt, Victoria, and Marcel were cofounders of the American AromaTherapy Association.

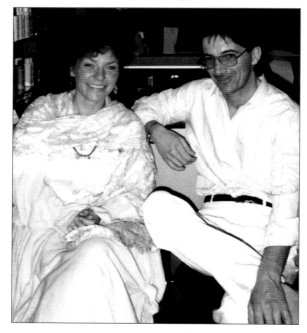

Marcel Lavabre and Colleen K. Dodt (author of The Essential Oils Book: Creating Personal Blends for Mind & Body *and* Natural Baby Care: Pure and Soothing Recipes and Techniques for Mothers and Babies)

aromatherapy produces 68,800,000 results. "Aromatherapy" products can be found in Walmart and practically every other big-box store that carries body-care products. Amazon offers hundreds of aromatherapy books and thousands of aromatherapy products by dozens of companies. And yes, you may have guessed it, there is an app for it—dozens of them actually, for both Android and Apple mobile devices. There are aromatherapy hash tags, Facebook groups, Pinterest pages, countless YouTube videos, and on and on. A TV series on the subject, titled *Everybody Nose,* was produced in 2007, with thirty-five episodes. Aromatherapy has been featured on everything from *The Oprah Winfrey Show* to *The Simpsons.* It is everywhere!

Grand View Research, a U.S.-based market research and consulting company, estimated the global aromatherapy market at $1.07 billion in 2016. Meanwhile, two major (and controversial) multilevel aromatherapy companies each claim to have broken $1 billion in yearly sales.

But aromatherapy is more than just another health fad or marketing trend. Aromatherapy is now used in hospitals in several European countries, including France, Germany, and the United Kingdom. In the U.K. hospitals have aromatherapists on staff, and aromatherapy is included in 90 percent of palliative care. In France pharmacies offer an extensive selection of essential oils, and aromatherapy is used in cancer care and geriatrics as a complementary treatment to improve quality of life for patients and to reduce anxiety and sleep disturbances.

In the United States the prestigious Mayo Clinic and many other hospitals offer aromatherapy care.

In Latin America my good friend, the unflagging Conie Bastar, has been preaching the aromatherapy gospel in Mexico for the past thirty years with her Instituto Mexicano de Aromaterapia. In 2001, Conie launched the Congreso Internacional de Aromaterapia with attendees from all over Latin America. Michael Scholes and I were guest speakers at the 2012, 2014, and 2017 congresses.

To my great surprise, Brazil appears to be the country where aromatherapy is most widely implemented in Latin America. It is, to my knowledge, the only country to celebrate a Dia da Aromaterapia (Aromatherapy Day), which happens to be on December 19, Gattefossé's birthday. The ministry of health approved the inclusion of aromatherapy in the Sistema Único de Saúde (SUS), the Brazilian public health care system, in early 2019. All public health clinics and doctors are now allowed to recommend aromatherapy to their patients.

The original *Aromatherapy Workbook* was launched at Aromatherapy 1990, the third aromatherapy congress of the American AromaTherapy Association, which featured all the major experts from the United States and Europe. I would never have dreamed that my humble workbook would still be in print thirty years later.

I felt humbled and honored when I was approached by the Laszlo Group in early 2018 with an invitation to be guest speaker at CIAROMA 2018, the third International

Aromatology Congress. I was thrilled when the Laszlo Group then offered to publish an updated edition of the *Aromatherapy Workbook* in Portuguese, just in time for that congress. The new Portuguese edition is greatly enhanced and augmented, with no less than three new chapters, including one on comparative study of the modes of administration of essential oils and an entire section on the art of blending. The Portuguese edition also includes lots of visual elements: pictures and graphics.

Having written all the updates to the Portuguese edition in English, an update to the U.S. edition was the logical next step. With the thirtieth anniversary of the original 1990 edition just around the corner, the publisher agreed to a Thirtieth Anniversary Edition that includes all the changes and additions to the Portuguese edition as well as a substantial rewriting of chapter 9, "The Essential Oils in Botanical Families." This chapter has been updated to reflect the enormous progress of botany over the past thirty years thanks to genetics and DNA mapping. It has been expanded and reordered. Each botanical family now includes photographs of its most characteristic elements. Additional visuals have been included throughout the entire book to make it more attractive and engaging.

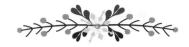

Acknowledgments

I thank the following people:

Jamaica Burns Griffin and her editorial team for their patience, dedication, suggestions, and relentless search for discrepancies, omissions, and potential misunderstanding. You all contributed to a much improved final version of this book.

Jean Valnet, one of the main pioneers of aromatherapy, who, with his book *The Practice of Aromatherapy,* contributed greatly to the revival of this art.

Robert Tisserand, who first spread the word in the English-speaking world.

Especially Henri Viaud, a French distiller from Provence who was the first to stress the importance of long, low-pressure distillation and the use of pure and natural essential oils from specified botanical origin and chemotypes and who has not always been credited for his contribution to aromatherapy. Viaud tried to distill practically everything that could be distilled. He was the first to produce and market oils such as St. John's wort and meadowsweet. He also revived the therapeutic use of floral waters. I learned a great deal from this wonderful *honête homme,* with his amazing and refreshing curiosity and eagerness for new experiments.

All humble producers who provide me with their oils.

Daniel Pénoël for his pioneering work in medical aromatherapy.

All those involved in the bettering and beautifying of our planetary village.

All my students throughout the world.

All the practitioners of the aromatic art.

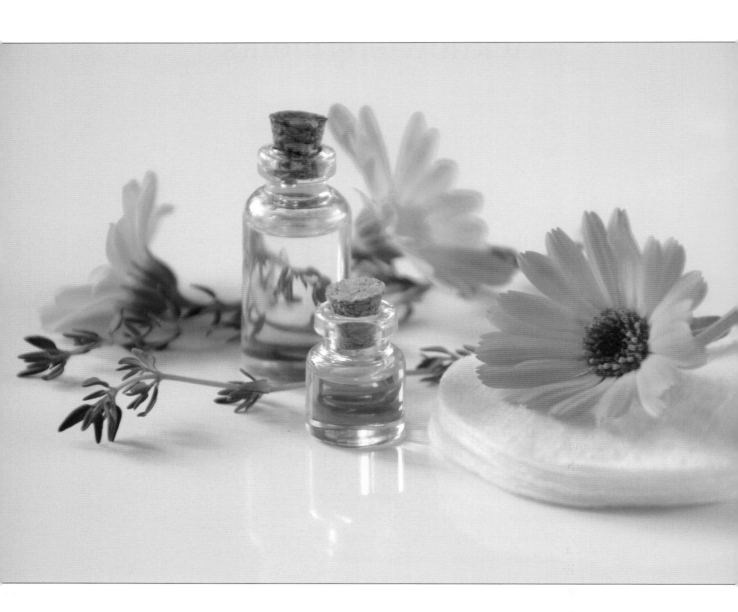

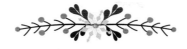

Introduction

Aromatherapy has known tremendous growth since this book was first published in 1990. It has now become a buzzword, used and abused by marketers and manufacturers of all types and credentials. The availability of essential oils and aromatherapy products has increased dramatically through all types of sources and distribution channels, from health food stores to spas and beauty salons and even department stores and pharmacies. Products with aromatherapy claims (but not much more) can be found in the mass market. With ever increasing media coverage and celebrities swearing by it, aromatherapy is more fashionable than ever.

But aromatherapy is not just a new trend, a new thing to do, as those who are involved in it can testify. In Europe, where it began more than sixty years ago, aromatherapy is practiced by medical doctors, nurses, and other health professionals. It is taught to medical students in France and is used by some English nurses in their hospitals. Extensive clinical research of aromatherapy is under way, mainly in these countries.

When people first hear about aromatherapy, they think about fragrance and perfumes, an alluring world of imagination, magic, and fantasy. But aromatherapy consists simply of using essential oils for healing.

Essential oils are volatile, oily substances; they are highly concentrated vegetal extracts that contain hormones, vitamins, antibiotics, and antiseptics. In a way, essential oils represent the spirit or soul of the plant. They are the most concentrated form of herbal energy. Many plants produce essential oils, which are contained in tiny droplets between cells and play an important role in the biochemistry of the plants. They are also responsible for the fragrance of the plants.

Essential oils are used in cosmetics and pharmacy as well as in perfumery. Their field of activity is quite wide, from deep therapeutic action to the extreme subtlety of genuine perfumes. In aromatherapy the essential oils can be taken internally in their pure form, diluted in alcohol, mixed with honey, or added in medical preparations. They are used externally in frictions (localized massage), massage, and olfactory exposure. Finally, they are ingredients of numerous cosmetics and perfumes.

Essential oils can have strictly allopathic effects (meaning that they act like regular medicines); more subtle effects, like those of Bach flower remedies of homeopathic preparations; and psychological and spiritual effects, which constitute their most traditional use. They are also powerful antiseptics and antibiotics that are not dangerous for the body. Aromatherapy is thus, in many cases, an excellent alternative to more aggressive therapies.

Essential oils are the "quintessences" of the alchemists. In this sense they condense the spiritual and vital forces of the plants in a material form; this power acts on the biological level to strengthen the natural defenses of the body and is the medium of a direct human–plant communication on the energetic and spiritual plane.

Aromatherapy can be used on many different levels. Essential oils are extremely versatile materials: they are both medicine and fragrance; they can cure the most severe physical condition and can reach to the depth of our souls.

Before you start reading this book, though, I warn you: once you step into the world of essences, you will be exposed to one of the most delightful and harmless forms of addiction. Chances are that you will want to know more and more about this amazing healing art. If you allow yourself to be touched by the power of these wonderful substances, you will discover a new world that is actually very old—the almost-forgotten world of nature's fragrances. This is a world without words, a world of images that you explore from the tip of your nose to the center of your brain—a world of subtle surprise and silent ecstasy.

ONE

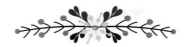

Aromatics and Perfumes in History

Since the earliest ages of humanity, aromatic fumigations have been used in daily rituals and during religious ceremonies as an expression and a reminder of an all-pervasive sacredness. Fragrance has been seen as a manifestation of divinity on earth, a connection between human beings and the gods, medium and mediator, emanation of matter and manifestation of spirit.

In a sense, the origins of aromatherapy can be traced back to the origins of humanity. Some anthropologists believe that the appearance of some form of rituals is the defining moment in the emergence of human culture. Since their origins, rituals have always involved fumigations and the burning of aromatic herbs and woods. Rituals were used mostly in healing ceremonies. What a great intuition! With the burning of aromatic substances, these fumigations diffuse essential oils, which have an antiseptic effect, into the air, bringing about physical healing. At the same time, the fragrance acts on a subtle level for psychic and spiritual healing.

AROMATIC MEDICINE IN EGYPT

The origin of aromatherapy is usually attributed to ancient Egypt and India. I would date it back to the fabulous and mysterious Kingdom of Sheba, located in the part of the world now called Ethiopia. Ethiopia is considered the cradle of humanity, where the most ancient remains of our distant ancestors have been found.

The Kingdom of Sheba, the "land of milk and honey," was a very prosperous country of high antiquity. In particular, it controlled the production of the very precious frankincense and myrrh and the trade in spices coming by caravan from India and then by boat through the Red Sea. Sheba is the land from where the three magi came to greet the infant Christ with gifts of gold, frankincense, and myrrh, the three most precious substances of the time.

There is also the fabulous story of the Queen of Sheba. While the Kingdom of Sheba

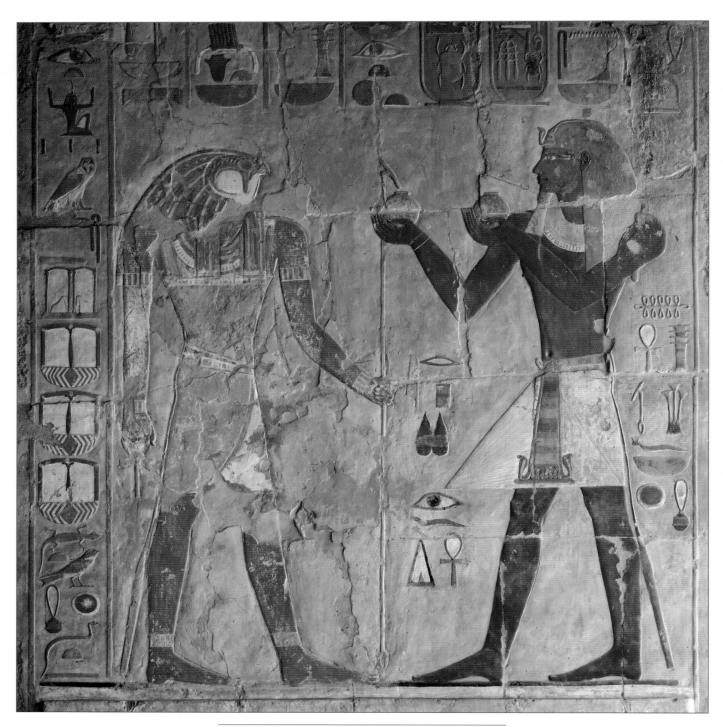

Aromatic medicine in Egypt

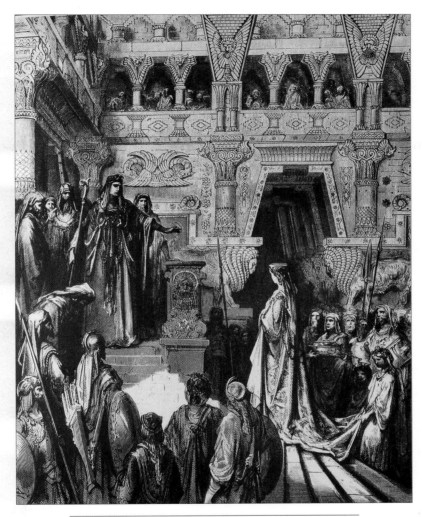

The Queen of Sheba visiting Solomon
by Gustave Doré, 1866

controlled the trade in frankincense and myrrh, the Queen of Sheba was doing a very hefty business with a tiny kingdom called Israel. Located at the outskirts of the known world, Israel was ruled by a king by the name of Solomon, whose fame had reached all the way to Sheba. The queen was known to be immensely rich, and Solomon had promised his god, Yahweh, to build a temple the likes of which had never been seen on the face of the earth. But the tiny kingdom was broke. Solomon sent emissaries to the queen, trying to borrow some gold from her. The queen was intrigued. She decided to undertake the perilous journey across the unforgiving desert to meet her client and potential debtor.

The queen was young and courageous, and her beauty was stunning. Solomon fell desperately in love with her at first sight. Under the spell of the queen's magnificent beauty, he neglected his wives and concubines, and even the governing of his kingdom. The queen eventually decided to return to her kingdom, bearing Solomon's child. Solomon never recovered from his lost love and tried to lose himself in debauchery. He also composed the very famous "Song of Songs," one of the most beautiful and erotic love poems in human literature.

There is evidence that the Egyptians borrowed some of their religious and political system from the land of Sheba. In Egypt medicine was inseparable from religion, and healing always took place in both body and mind. The use of perfumes and aromatics was originally a privilege of the pharaohs and the high priests. The priests developed a very sophisticated pharmacy, using large quantities of aromatics, which were also used for the preparation and preservation of mummies. The Egyptians made extensive use of substances such as myrrh and frankincense, as well as rose and jasmine. These products were so precious that they were traded as currency.

The Egyptians are considered the inventors of Western medicine, pharmacy, and cosmetology. Parallel with the development of medicine and pharmacy, they also developed very refined techniques for skin care, creating beauty recipes that have endured to the present day. Aromatics were the major active ingredients in their skin care preparations. Cleopatra, of course, is legendary for her use of cosmetic preparations and perfumes to enhance her beauty and her powers of seduction. When she sailed to greet the Roman emperor Marc Antony, the sails of her ship were soaked in jasmine, one of the most aphrodisiac fragrances. Marc Antony fell so deeply in love with Cleopatra that he gave up his empire to follow her.

Aromatic medicine emerged from the shade of smoky temples in Egypt—the birthplace of medicine, perfumery, and pharmacy—more than six thousand years ago. The precious substances came from all parts of the world, carried by caravan or by boat: cedar from Lebanon; roses from Syria; and spikenard, myrrh, frankincense, labdanum, and cinnamon from Babylon, Ethiopia, Somalia, and even Persia and India.

The priest supervised the preparations in the temples, reading the formulas and chanting incantations, while the students mixed the ingredients. Pulverization, maceration, and other operations could continue for months until the right subtle fragrance was obtained for ceremonial use.

But spiritual matters were not the only concern of the Egyptians. They attached the greatest importance to health and hygiene and were thoroughly familiar with the effect of perfumes and aromatic substances on the body and the psyche. Many preparations were used for both their fragrant quality and their healing power. Kephi, for example, a perfume of universal fame, was an antiseptic, a balsamic, and a tranquilizer that could be taken internally.

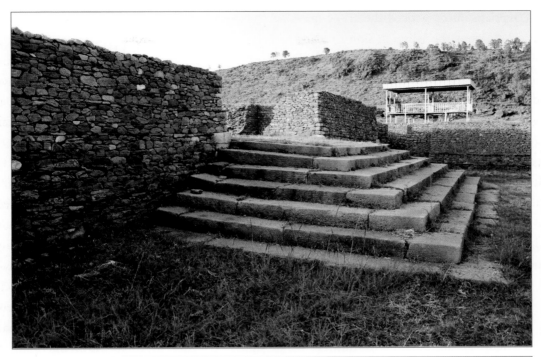

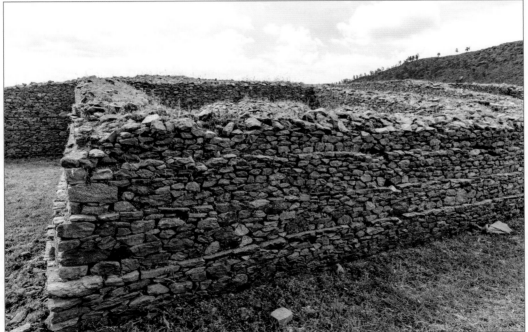

Ruins of Queen of Sheba's palace, Aksum, Ethiopia

The Egyptians also practiced the art of massage and were famous specialists in skin care and cosmetology. Their products were renowned all over the civilized world. The Phoenician merchants exported Egyptian unguents, scented oils, creams, and aromatic wines all over the Mediterranean world and the Arabic peninsula and thereby enhanced the fame and wealth of Egypt.

Embalming was one of the main uses of aromatics. Bodies were filled with perfumes, resins, and fragrant preparations after removal of the internal organs. So strong is the antiseptic power of essential oils that the tissues are still well preserved thousands of years later. In the seventeenth century mummies were sold in Europe, and doctors distilled them and used them as ingredients in numerous medicines. The use of aromatics spread from Egypt to Israel, Greece, Rome, and the whole Mediterranean world. Every culture and civilization, from the most primitive to the most sophisticated, developed its own practice of perfumery and cosmetics.

India is probably the only place in the world where this tradition was never lost. With more than ten thousand years of continuous practice, Ayurvedic medicine is the oldest continuous form of medical practice. The Vedas, the most sacred books of India and among the oldest known books, mention more than seven hundred different products, such as cinnamon, spikenard, coriander, ginger, myrrh, and sandalwood. The Vedas codify the uses of perfumes and aromatics for liturgical and therapeutic purpose.

DISTILLATION AND ALCHEMY

In Europe the advent of Christianity and the fall of the Roman Empire marked the beginning of a long period of barbarism and a general decline of all knowledge. Revival came from the Arabic countries with the birth of Islam. Intellectual and cultural activity flourished, as did the arts. Arabic civilization attained an unequaled degree of refinement. The philosophers devoted themselves to the old hermetic art of alchemy, whose origin was attributed to the Egyptian god Tehuti. They renewed the use of aromatics in medicine and perfumery and perfected the techniques. The great philosopher Avicenna invented the refrigerated coil, a real breakthrough in the art of distillation.

Alchemy, which was probably introduced to Europe by the Crusaders on their way back from the Holy Land, was primarily a spiritual quest, and the different operations performed by the adept were symbolic of the processes taking place within the alchemist. Distillation was the symbol of purification and the concentration of spiritual forces.

In the alchemist's vision, everything, from sand and stones to plants and people, was made up of a physical body, a soul, and a spirit. In accordance with the basic principle of *solve* and *coagula* (dissolve and coagulate), the art of *spagyrie* consisted of dissolving the physical body and condensing the soul and spirit, which had all the curative power, into the quintessences. The material was distilled over and over to remove all impurities, and the final products were highly potent medicines.

With the expansion of this mysterious art, more and more substances were processed for the extraction of essences. These quintessences were the basis of most medicines, and for centuries essential oils remained the only remedies for epidemic diseases.

THE RENAISSANCE, DECLINE, AND REBIRTH

During the Renaissance the use of essential oils expanded into perfumery and cosmetics. With further progress in the arts of chemistry and distillation, the production of elixirs, balms, scented waters, fragrant oils, and unguents for medicine and skin care flourished. Nicholas Lemery, the personal physician of Louis XIV, described many such preparations in the *Dictionnaire des drogues simples.* Some have survived until now: melissa water, arquebuse water, and the famous Cologne water, for instance, are still produced.

The arrival of modern science in the nineteenth century marked the decline of all forms of herbal therapy. The early scientists had a simplistic and somewhat naive vision of the world. When the first plant alkaloids were discovered, scientists thought it better to keep only the main active principals of the plants and then reproduce them in laboratories. Thus they discovered and reproduced penicillin (from a natural mold growing on bread), aspirin (naturally present in birch, wintergreen, and meadowsweet), antibiotics, and so on.

Without denying the obvious value of many scientific discoveries, we must acknowledge that the narrow vision of the allopathic medical profession has led to some abuses. Microorganisms adapt to antibiotics much faster than does the human body, making antibiotics inefficient as well as dangerous to the body. Corticosteroids have dreadful side effects; hypnotics, antidepressants, and amphetamines are highly addictive; and so on.

THE BIRTH OF MODERN AROMATHERAPY: AROMATHERAPY IN FRANCE

Aromatherapy per se was formally developed in France in the late 1920s and grew into a mainstream movement in Europe. The term itself was coined by a French chemist by the name of René-Maurice Gattefossé. As the story goes, Mr. Gattefossé, who was a chemist working for the perfume industry, burned his hand in an explosion in his laboratory. A vat full of lavender oil was nearby, and he plunged his hand into it. The pain disappeared instantly, and he recovered so fast that he decided to investigate further the healing power of essential oils. Thus was born modern aromatherapy.

I personally have experienced the quasi-miraculous effect of lavender oil on burns on several occasions. A few years ago, while cooking asparagus in a pressure cooker, I spilled more than half a gallon of boiling water on my feet and legs. I removed my socks promptly and applied lavender neat on the whole area

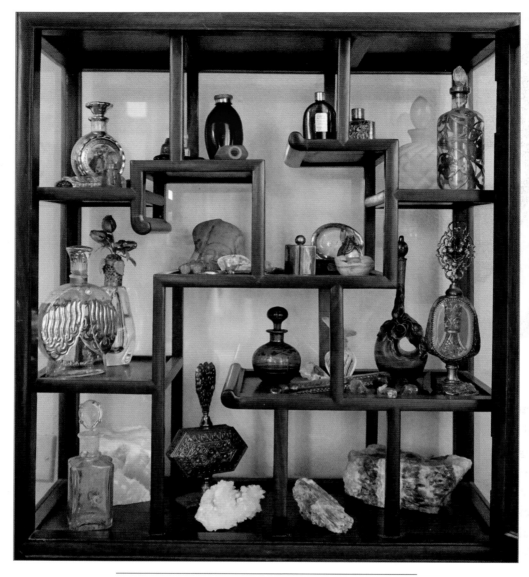

Author's personal collection of perfume bottles

and continued applying it every ten to fifteen minutes for a few hours. Not only did the pain disappear, but I never blistered or lost skin! Likewise, when my daughter was twelve years old she fell asleep on the beach on a very hot summer day. She had forgotten to use any sunscreen, and the Southern California sun was implacable. She came home redder than a lobster. I instantly applied to her face and body an oil that contains lavender,

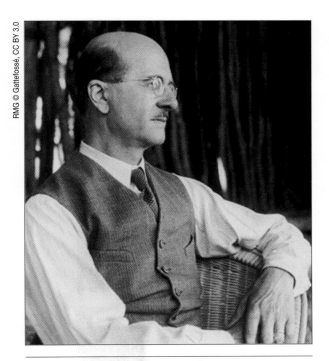

René-Maurice Gattefossé, 1940s

contributed to the popularity of aromatherapy in the 1960s and '70s. The major figures of the 1980s and '90s were the conservative Drs. Lapraz, Belaiche, and Duraffourd—defenders of medical orthodoxy—on the one hand; and Pierre Franchomme, a creative but controversial pioneer, who struck gold in the '90s when he was hired by Estée Lauder to create the "Origins" line. A former Franchomme associate, Dr. Daniel Pénoël, also started working on his own to develop his special techniques on the basis of "live embalming," a massage of the body with pure essential oils.

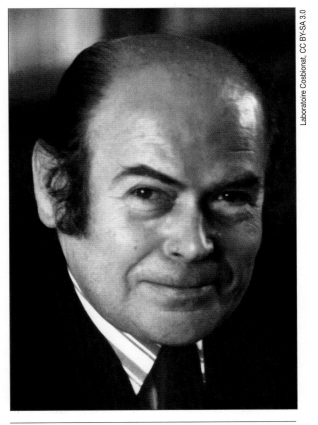

Jean Valnet (1920–1995)

marjoram, and neroli in an oil base of sweet almond, hazelnut, and vitamin E. I continued applying it every hour for the first evening and then twice a day for a few days. Again, my daughter didn't blister or peel.

Back to the 1920s the curative power of essential oils was well known, and many essential oils belonged to the European pharmacopoeia (and still do), which means that they are classified as active medical ingredients.

The French emphasized the medical uses of aromatherapy and conducted extensive research on the antiseptic and antibiotic use of essential oils. Aromatherapy is taught in medical schools and is practiced by medical doctors and naturopaths. Dr. Jean Valnet widely

The French have developed the skin care uses of aromatherapy since the 1980s and '90s. French aestheticians have grown increasingly attracted to aromatherapy, thanks mostly to lines like Decléor. The French in general, even in the skin care area, tend to use much higher dosages and concentrations than do other European practitioners. Preparations with 10 percent essential oils are not unheard of for professional products, resulting in products that must be used with extreme caution by highly trained professionals. Essential oils and aromatherapy products can be found in all health food stores and many pharmacies and have a stable following. Still, aromatherapy in France has never made headlines the way it has in the United States or the United Kingdom.

The European aromatherapy market evolved in various countries along quite different lines, with each country developing one specific area of application. Only now do we see some overlapping of the various approaches.

British aromatherapy began in the 1950s with Marguerite Maury, a French cosmetologist who lived in London and emphasized uses in skin care and massage, with an esoteric undercurrent. She gave British aromatherapy the spiritualist undertones that it still retains.

The major figures in the United Kingdom are Robert Tisserand, Patricia Davis, Shirley Price, and Valerie Worwood. Aromatherapy has become extremely popular in the United Kingdom since the late 1980s, when it was known that its adepts included Ms. Thatcher and the royal family, from Princess Diana and

Fergie to Prince Charles. The royals are still patrons of aromatherapy; Meghan Markle swears by tea tree oil. She had the walls of the nursery painted with rosemary-infused vegan paint to welcome baby Archie Harrison Mountbatten-Windsor.

Aromatherapy is now a well-developed movement in the United Kingdom, and nurses are helping it expand in the health fields; a group of dedicated nurses gives aromatherapy massage to patients in British hospitals.

If the French can be somewhat reckless, the British tend to be overly cautious. Dosages rarely exceed a few drops per ounce. Their list of contraindications seems to be growing by the day, with no scientific or anecdotal evidence to sustain it. As pointed out by a frustrated aromatherapist in a recent debate on the subject, there is still not one single reported accident involving essential oils in the United Kingdom.

Curiously, Europeans have yet to really discover the effect of essential oils as fragrances. Americans, on the other hand, tend to see aromatherapy as the use of fragrances for their mood-enhancing effects, which after all is the most obvious effect of essential oils.

AROMATHERAPY IN THE UNITED STATES

Aromatherapy did not exist in any significant way in the United States until the early 1980s. In fact, when I first moved here in 1981, aromatherapy was still virtually unknown.

The aromatherapy movement in the United States can be separated into two very different approaches: a genuine approach and a mass-market approach. Genuine aromatherapy is education driven and aims at achieving a synthesis of the various approaches of aromatherapy, which have flourished primarily in Europe. This approach is based on the study of essential oils as chemical substances as well as fragrances. It integrates the various effects of essential oils as healing and curative agents for the body with their properties on the energetic and mental levels. Genuine aromatherapy aims to develop practical techniques that integrate the various effects of the oils in a synergistic way. It encompasses body care, skin care, and massage and touches every aspect of daily life. It is part of a natural way of life, an *art de vivre,* that integrates body, mind, and spirit and is geared more toward maintaining health than curing diseases.

Interest in genuine aromatherapy has been growing steadily over the years and is now booming exponentially. The spa, massage, and skin care markets, as well as the health food market, are the most receptive to the concept.

Mass marketers are always looking for the next new trend, and with aromatherapy, they may have found a cash cow. This has given birth to a rather reduced and oversimplified version of aromatherapy, focusing on the uses of fragrances (and not necessarily natural essential oils) for their mood-enhancing properties.

Americans are without a doubt mass-marketing geniuses, but the contribution of Coca-Cola and McDonald's to the fine art of cuisine is questionable, to say the least. While aromatherapy is now under the spotlight of the mass media, receiving intense coverage, there is a danger that it might very well be emptied of its substance in the process. However, the media and the public in general are much more sophisticated today than they ever were. We can hope that genuine aromatherapy will take advantage of the momentum created by mass media to promote the real thing.

TWO

Aromatherapy
A Multilevel Therapy

SCIENTIFIC RESEARCH AND MODERN AROMATHERAPY

Modern aromatherapy was born in the early twentieth century with the works of the French chemist R. M. Gattefossé and attracted interest in France, Germany, Switzerland, and Italy—and later on in the United States in the 1980s. Many studies have been conducted by laboratory scientists and by practicing therapists. Most of this research, somewhat constrained by the dominant scientific ideology, almost exclusively concerns the antiseptic and antibiotic powers of essential oils and their allopathic properties.

Since the early 1980s, however, in part thanks to the work of Dr. Schwartz at Yale University and of professors Dodd and Van Toller at Warwick University in England, a better understanding of the mechanisms of olfaction has opened new, exciting avenues for research and experimentation in aromatherapy.

The Antiseptic Power of Essential Oils

After Pasteur, belief in external agents (microbes, spores, viruses) as the cause of diseases became the basic assumption of official medicine. It was natural, in this context, that the first studies of essential oils should concern their antiseptic properties. Koch himself studied the action of turpentine on *Bacillus anthracis* in 1881; in 1887, Chamberland studied the action of the essential oils of oregano, cinnamon, and clove buds. Other studies by Rideal and Walker and Kellner and Kober proposed different methods of measuring the antiseptic power of essential oils in direct contact or in their vaporized states.

The Aromatogram

With the aromatogram, Dr. Maurice Girault went one step further and provided a useful tool for prescription and diagnosis. Girault, a French gynecologist and obstetrician, studied the effects of essential oils and tinctures (in association with other natural therapies—homeopathy, minerals, etc.) in gynecology for years. The results of his work were published in *Traité de Phytothérapie et d'Aromatherapie,* Volume 3, *Gynecologie* (Belaiche and Girault, 1979).

In the aromatogram, vaginal secretions on a swab are tested against several essential oils to determine which oil is the most efficient against the specific microorganism. This method was extended to all infectious disease by French aromatherapy doctors Pradal, Belaiche, Andou, and Durrafourd. It had the advantage of dealing with real germs coming from real sites in real patients, rather than from laboratories.

VIRTUALLY NO RESISTANCE PHENOMENA

For all their imperfections and limitations, the various methods of analyzing the germicidal power of essential oils have given scientific validation to aromatherapy. The action of essences on microorganisms is now better understood: essences inhibit certain metabolic functions of microorganisms, such as growth and multiplication, eventually destroying them if the inhibition continues.

Even though there is general agreement on the antiseptic power of essential oils, different authors classify them differently by their antigenetic properties. Since essential oils are products of life, their chemical composition depends on so many factors that it is impossible to obtain exactly the same essence twice. Therefore different analyses will give different results. According to Jean Valnet, microorganisms show no resistance to essential oils. Recent research on the subject suggests that resistance occurs, but to a far lesser degree than to synthetic antibiotics. This makes sense, as essential oils have a more complex structure and moreover are produced by the defense mechanisms of the plant.

The Power of Living Substances

The real interest of essential oils in medicine lies in their action on the site. Even if they could easily and advantageously be replaced by synthetic products for their antiseptic uses, these synthetics would always be awkward in their interaction with the body as a whole, even though synthetics are chemical reconstructions of components naturally occurring in essential oils.

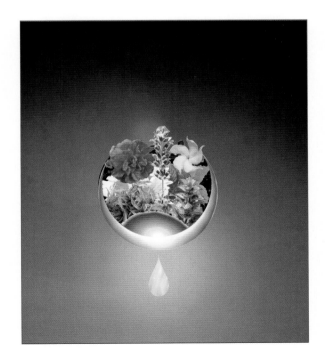

Essential oils have hundreds of chemical components, most of them in very small amounts. We know that certain trace elements are fundamental for life. In the same way, the power of living products lies in the combination of their elements, and their trace components are at least as important as their main components. No synthetic reconstruction can fully replicate a natural product. It is thus very important to always use natural essential oils.

A HOLISTIC PERSPECTIVE

The human body is a whole, and the interactions taking place among the whole, its parts, and the environment are regulated according to a principle of equilibrium called homeostasis. Homeostasis is an autoregulation process that is ensured by substances such as hormones and the secretions of endocrine glands controlled by the corticohypothalamo-hypophyseal complex. Any external or internal aggression brings a compensatory regulation (hyper- or hypofunctioning) and an imbalance that provokes a defense reaction; the ingestion of chemicals often creates such an imbalance. In disease, chemotherapy consists of answering one aggression with another, creating a state of war highly prejudicial to the battleground—the human body!

We depend on plants in every domain—food, energy, and oxygen—and there is between plants and humans a complementary relationship. We are part of the same whole, which is life itself. This is why plants are not aggressive to the body. (Only abuse of plants can be aggressive.)

Hippocrates, the father of occidental medicine, founded his practice on two basic principles: the principles of similarities (treat the same with the same, the poison with the poison) and the principle of oppositions (find antidotes). The latter, quite straightforward in its application, is the basis of modern medicine (allopathy). The former requires intuition and subtlety; it inspired the theory of similarities as formulated by the great alchemist and philosopher Paracelsus in the Middle Ages. It is also the basic principle of homeopathy and anthroposophic medicine.

From observing the morphology of plants and their different characteristics (their taste, their scent, the environment and soil in which they grow, and their overall vibration), Paracelsus could predict their therapeutic indications. Rudolf Steiner and the anthroposophists adopted the same methods. Their findings have been amazingly accurate and have been largely confirmed by scientific research.

Theories of information and genetics, dealing with the issues of order and chaos, give further justification to such an approach. According to these theories, adaptability and mobility in the use of information are among the chief characteristics of life. A living system (a cell, an organism, a colony of insects, a social group) starts with a certain range of potentials that become actual in a feedback process with the environment. Thus the embryo and the human being develop from a single primordial cell by differentiation. Life, on the other hand, apparently uses universal structures (such as chromosomic or enzymatic structures). Living systems seem able to "borrow" information from other living systems; to some extent, they are able to incorporate alien information.

If the clue to recovery lies within oneself, it should be very beneficial to give the right kind of information to the body. Therefore close investigation of the role of essential oils in plants will help us understand their curative power, while the observation of specific plants will tell us about the healing properties of each individual oil.

Essential oils evidently play a key role in the biochemistry of the plants; they are like the hormones contained in small "bags" located between the cells, and they act as regulators and messengers. They catalyze biochemical reactions, protect the plant from parasites and diseases, and play an important role in fertilization. (Orchids, the most fascinating family of plants, have developed this process to a high degree, attracting the most suitable insects to carry precious pollen to their remote sexual partners.)

Essential oils carry information between the cells and are related to the hormonal response of the plant to stressful situations. They are agents of the plant's adaptation to its environment. It is not surprising, then, that they contain hormones. Sage, traditionally known to regulate and promote menstruation, contains estrogen. Ginseng, a well-known tonic and aphrodisiac, contains substances similar to estrone. Estrogens can also be found in parsley, hops, and licorice. Rosemary increases the secretion of bile and facilitates its excretion.

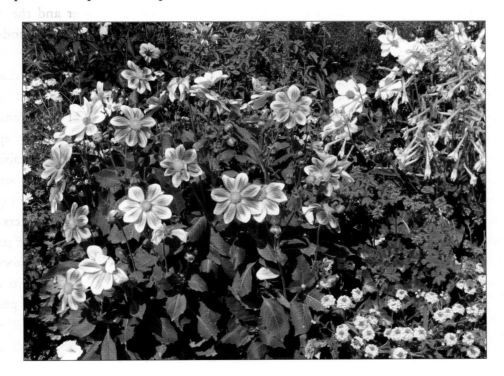

Essential oils control the multiplication and renewal of cells. They have cytophilactic and healing effects on the human body (especially lavender, geranium, garlic, hyssop, and sage). According to Jean Valnet, they have anticarcinogenic properties. They are often present in the outer part of leaves, in the skin of citrus fruits, and in the bark of certain trees. Cosmetic applications are among their oldest uses.

Most aromatic plants grow in dry areas, and the essential oils in them are produced by solar activity. In the anthroposophic vision, essential oils are the manifestation of the cosmic fire forces. They are produced by the plant's cosmic self. In them, matter dissolves into warmth. Therefore they are indicated for diseases originating in the astral body.

AROMATICS AND THE SOUL

Aromatherapy acts at different levels. There is first an allopathic action due to the chemical composition of the essential oils and their antiseptic, stimulant, calming, antineuralgic, or other properties. There is a more subtle action at the level of information, similar to the action of homeopathic or anthropsophic remedies. Last but not least, essential oils act on the mind. In fact they are most traditionally used as basic ingredients of perfumes. Generally speaking, pleasant odors have obvious uplifting effects. According to Marguerite Maury in *The Secret of Life and Youth:*

Of the greatest interest is the effect of fragrances on the psychic and mental state of the individual. Power of perception becomes clearer and more acute, and there is a feeling of having, to a certain extent, outstripped events. . . . It might even be said that the emotional trouble which in general obscures our perception is practically suppressed.

Anatomy of Olfaction

Research conducted in Europe, the United States, and the former Soviet Union reveals that the effects of odors on the psyche may be more important than scientists have suspected. The University of Warwick, England, has conducted fascinating research on this subject (see Theimer, *Fragrance Chemistry: The Science of the Sense of Smell*). Figure 2.1 illustrates the anatomy of olfaction.

The sense of smell acts mostly on a subconscious level; the olfactory nerves are directly connected to the most primitive part of the brain, the limbic system—our connection with our remote saurian ancestors, our distant reptile cousins. In a sense, the olfactory nerve is an extension of the brain itself, which can then be reached directly through the nose. This is the only such open gate to the brain.

The limbic system, originally known as the rhinecephalon ("smell brain"), is the part of the brain that regulates the sensorimotor activity and deals with the primitive drives of sex, hunger, and thirst. Stimulation of the olfactory bulb sends electrical signals to the area of the limbic system concerned with visceral and behavioral mechanisms; they directly affect the digestive and sexual systems and emotional behavior. In

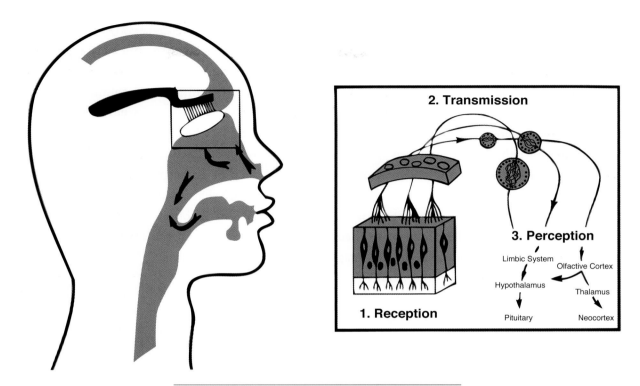

Fig. 2.1. The anatomy of olfaction

fact, the brain's electrical response to odors is about the same as the one correlated with emotions. (In the French language the same verb, *sentir,* is used for "to smell" and "to feel.") The processes of olfactory reception are largely unconscious; we are mostly unaware of our scent environment. For some yet-unexplained reason, whenever we are in contact with a new odor we lose our consciousness of it after a while. The electrical signals correlated to this odor still continue to reach the brain, but the contacts with our conscious centers have been shut off. This shows how little control our conscious centers have on the olfactory stimulations.

The sense of smell is very sensitive: we can detect up to 1 part of fragrant material in 10,000 billion parts or more. A trained nose can differentiate several hundred different odors. However, we have no proper vocabulary to talk about odors. We say that something smells like a rose, strawberry, skunk, or whatever. The olfactory nerves terminate in a part of the brain that does not use the same kind of logic as our intellectual centers. Although odors form a kind of communication system, they cannot be developed as a language; they work through associations and images and are not analytical.

In *Perfumery: The Psychology and Biology of Fragrance* (Van Toller and Dodd, eds.), E. Douek describes various olfactory abnormalities. According to the author, anosmia, the total inability to smell, is always accompanied by some elements of depression, which can often become severe. With loss of the sense of smell, people also lose the sense of taste. The world becomes dull and colorless.

Even more interesting is parosmia, or olfactory illusion (usually related to a perception of bad odors). In such cases shy and withdrawn people tend to feel that the unpleasant odors they perceive emanate from themselves, while people with paranoid tendencies perceive them as coming from others. The latter suspect imaginary plots in their associates and generally show tyrannical tendencies. According to Douek, the French king Louis XI suffered from this affliction. He was very good at filling up his prisons and inventing sophisticated tortures to obtain confessions from his victims. It might be instructive to investigate the olfactory sanity of the most prominent tyrants throughout history!

Olfactory System and Sexual Mechanisms

Mammals release sexual olfactory signals called pheromones through specialized scent-producing apocrine glands. In humans, most of these glands are located in the circumanal and anogenital region, the chest and the abdomen, and around the nipples, with some variations between the different races.

D. M. Stoddart notes in *Perfumery: The Psychology and Biology of Fragrance* (Van Toller and Dodd, eds.) that most perfumes contain ingredients that mimic these sexual olfactory signals, such as civet, musk, or castoreum, and also substances like sandalwood (remarkably similar, according to the author, to androsterol, a male human pheromone). According to G. H. Dodd, humans secrete musklike molecules, and therefore we experience this type of odor in utero, which could explain the universal liking for it. The main function of perfumes would then be to heighten and fortify natural odors, rather than to cover them. The connection between olfaction and the sexual system takes place through the hypothalamic region. According to Stoddart:

> The hypothalamic region is a major receiver of olfactory neurons, and releases a variety of . . . hormones which pass to the anterior pituitary via the hypophyseal portal system, and induces the pituitary to secrete the suite of hormones which governs and controls the mammalian sexual cycles.

The synchronization of menstrual periods in girls' boarding schools is a well-known phenomenon. Several studies have shown that such synchronicity could be caused by axillary secretions (i.e., by pheromones).

In another now famous experiment, set up in a kindergarten, children playing near a pile of T-shirts worn by their mothers could accurately find their own mother's T-shirt within a very short time. Most of them would then retire to a corner with the T-shirt and quiet down. Although this experiment is not directly concerned with sexual matters, it shows the strong olfactory component of the mother–infant bond. It is also worth noting that breastfed babies develop a much stronger olfactory bond to their mother than do bottlefed ones.

The Gate to the Soul

When Sigmund Freud opened the Pandora's box of the unconscious at the beginning of this century, he suspected sexual drives to be the central feature of the show being played on our private stage. He considered the repression of smell to be a major cause of mental illness and suspected that the nose was related to the sexual organs. (Allergy to odors is a psychosomatic disease.)

If psychoanalysis and its avatars are to explore the unconscious from the mental side, the nose and the sense of smell give access to Pandora's box from the other side: the unknown side, the saurian side, from the origin of ages. The subtle emanations create a diffuse network that connects us to the unconscious of species, and to life itself. The strongest and deepest experiences are often accompanied by olfactory sensations. All traditions, even the most puritan, have known the power of fragrances; every religion knew their ceremonial use (usually in connection with sounds and colors) to generate elation among the faithful. Mystics or visionaries experience heavenly fragrances in their deepest ecstasy. Such people may eventually die in the "odor of sanctity."

Fragrances can bring about the deepest but most fugitive sensations. Like happiness, or love, or laughter, they catch you, almost by surprise, and fade away as soon as you try to grasp them. As you walk along the street, pull out the weeds in your backyard, hike on a trail, or sip your coffee, a mysterious emanation suddenly strikes your nose and the magic unfolds. In an instant of rapture, waves of delight run through your entire body, bringing about images and new sensations. But if you try to analyze what is going on, the experience disappears like a soap bubble; if you try to talk about it, you will soon fall short of words.

According to Jean-Jacques Rousseau, the sense of smell is imagination itself. Some authors needed olfactory sensations to stimulate their creativity. Guy de Maupassant, for instance, used to soak strawberries in a bowl of ether. Friedrich von Schiller filled the top drawer of his desk with overly ripe apples.

The sense of smell is closely related to memory; olfactory memories are very accurate and almost indelible. A French psychoanalyst, André Virel, used fragrance to bring forth hidden memories. The odor and taste of a madeleine dipped in a cup of tea inspired Marcel Proust to write one of the most remarkably precise and vivid works of introspection, a masterpiece of literature.

We probably all have our own private madeleines. Syringa, to me, is one of the most heavenly fragrances. It transports me to a space of undisturbed peacefulness where I can vividly recall the vegetable garden of my early childhood, with its fallen trellis, its dry wall above the dirt road leading to the spring, and its basin of fresh running water. There is a huge fig tree in the corner just above the road and a stone shed, falling in ruins on the other side, with a bush of syringa in the middle. I am leaning against the bush now in full bloom; I have been here for hours. Out there, behind the stone arch, is the farm, and then the world. But here, the warm and gentle sun of May envelops my frail body; the divine fragrance of syringa bathes my soul. I am totally at home. Why should I ever move?

PSYCHOTHERAPY AND AROMATHERAPY: A WIDE OPEN FIELD

Since the olfactory system is such an open gate to the subconscious, one would expect that psychotherapy could benefit from the use of olfactory stimuli for the cure of psychological disorders. Very little research has been done in this area, however, possibly because it is hard to systematize any kind of therapeutic procedure. The sense of smell is very private. Each individual's associations are different. Dr. A. D. Armond, for instance, reported the case of an anxious patient who worked on motorbikes and kept an oily washer in his pocket for comfort in times of stress.

Still, aromatherapy can offer some valuable tools to the practitioner. Oils such as neroli, lavender, marjoram, rose, and ylang-ylang have been traditionally used for their calming effects in stress reduction. Jasmine is a wonderful uplifting oil for the treatment of depression or anxiety, and there are many more (see chapter 8 and appendices 1 and 2). Diffusion is probably one of the best methods of using essential oils in this way.

One procedure often used by therapists is to prepare an appropriate blend of oils to use during the therapeutic session. The patient can then use the same blend at home to further the treatment. This method is particularly efficient when used in conjunction with any technique conducive to deep relaxation (such as hypnosis, meditation, yoga, or certain types of massage), as the olfactory stimuli are then more likely to have a deep impact on the patient.

Obviously psychoaromatherapy (a term coined by Robert Tisserand) is still a wide-open field in which experimentation should be encouraged. With minimal caution, no adverse side effects can be expected from the use of aroma in psychotherapy, while the potential benefits appear to be unlimited. I am personally very curious about any finding in this fascinating domain and invite my therapist readers to share their experience in this area with me.

UN JE NE SAIS QUOI, UN PRESQUE RIEN

Essential oils and fragrances have been extensively used for well-being—one of the main keys to health—since the beginning of civilization. Vladimir Jankelevitch, a French philosopher who gave cooking classes to his delighted students in the venerable Sorbonne, talked about *un je ne sais quoi, un presque rien* ("an I-don't-know-what, an almost-nothing") to characterize the subtle quality of an *art de vivre,* which can be extended to the basic jubilation of just being alive. This *je ne sais quoi,* this *presque rien* that is the mark of genuine art, of elegance, of humor, which differentiates a real meal from a mere quantity of proteins, calories, vitamins, and minerals, describes perfectly the contribution of fragrances to the quality of life. It is unpredictable, it cannot be analyzed by any scientific method, and yet it can be experienced. According to Goethe, the most evolved plants go through a transformation from the primitive germ to the exuberance of the flower in a natural movement toward spirituality in which the flower, in its impermanence and openness, represents an instant of rapture and jubilation. Fragrance is a manifestation of this jubilation.

Fragrances have their own language. Better than any word, they can express the most subtle feelings. Much is revealed about a person by his or her choice of fragrance and how that fragrance reacts with the skin. Everyone has his or her specific odor, which changes depending on the physical and mental state of the individual; thus, dogs can find lost people and criminals. Smell may, in fact, be a determinant in the establishment of relationships. It has also been a traditional tool for diagnosis (each disease is said to have its specific odor).

Aromas, even if they cannot change an individual, may help to create a positive groundwork if properly chosen. Fragrances stimulate the dynamic and positive aspect of the being by an effect of resonance. During the Renaissance the grande dames had their own secret perfumes; numerous systems associate perfumes with astrological signs, dominant planets, or morphological characteristics.

In conclusion, even though it can relieve symptoms, aromatherapy primarily aims at curing the causes of diseases. The main therapeutic action of essential oils consists in strengthening the organs and their functions and acting on the defense mechanism of the body. They do not do the job for the body; they help the body do its own job and thus do not weaken the organism. Their action is enhanced by all natural therapies that aim to restore the vitality of the individual. Maurice Girault recommended using them in conjunction with minerals, homeopathy, and psychotherapy. To this list I add nutrition, as food is the basis of animal life; depending on its quality, food can be the best medicine or the main cause of disease.

THREE

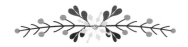

Essential Oils

Extraction and Adulteration

ESSENTIAL OILS IN THE PLANT

Essential oils are the fragrant principle of the plant. They are the chemical components that give a plant its characteristic fragrance.

In the spiritualistic approach to aromatherapy, essential oils are considered the life force, the energy of the plant. Alchemists regard them as the quintessence, the soul, the spirit of the plant. Anthroposophists see them as

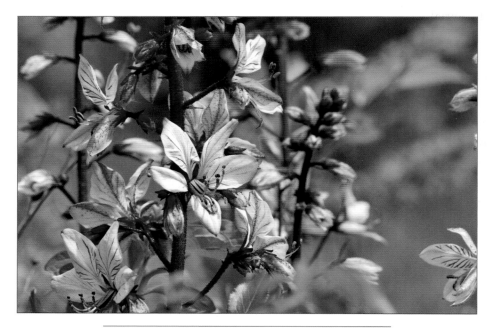

Dictamnus, *burning bush*

produced through the action of astral forces in the plant.

Essential oils are a type of vegetal hormone that helps the plant in its adaptation to the environment. From a biochemical point of view, they can be considered part of the plant's immune system. In extreme climates, such as the Arabian desert, certain plants use essential oils as a protection against the sun. Myrrh and frankincense bushes are surrounded by a very thin cloud of essential oils, which filters the sun's rays and freshens the air around the bushes. *Dictamnus fraxinella,* a plant of the same family that grows in the Sinai, is so literally endowed with resinous oil glands that the resinous vapor perpetually surrounding the shrub burns with a brilliant glow when lit. (According to Roy Genders, the burning bush that Moses saw in the Sinai could have been caused by such a phenomenon.) Essential oils also protect the plant from diseases and parasites.

The plant uses essential oils from its flowers for its reproductive process. It attracts specific insects by releasing fragrances that mimic the insect's pheromones to facilitate pollination. In a way, essential oils from flowers are part of the plant's sexual system. We describe many essential oils that have aphrodisiac properties and other properties that relate to reproduction and sexuality (emmenagogues, hormone balancers, PMS or menopause relief, etc.).

Certain essential oils have the power to repel insects that could be harmful to the plant. For example, citronella and geranium are mosquito repellent and lavender and spike repel

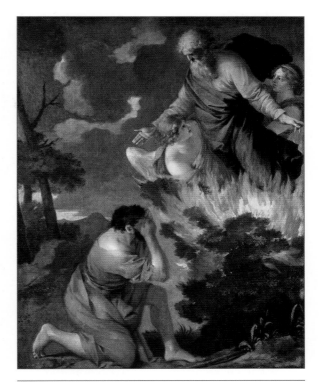

Moses and the Burning Bush *by Sébastien Bourdon (1616–1671)*

fleas and mites. They sometimes even act as natural selective weedkillers, creating a territory around their roots where certain other plants cannot grow. Organic and biodynamic farmers know how to take advantage of this phenomenon in their work: certain plants have dynamic effects on the growth of specific plants while inhibiting others.

The plant stores its essential oils in small pouches. It is important to note that plants do not use essential oils in their pure form. Plants store essential oils in specific areas and retrieve them in a diluted form when they are needed for the plant's biochemical processes. Humans, like plants, should not use essential oils in their pure form. Do not try to be smarter than plants!

Essential oils are usually located on the outer part of the plant. They can be seen on the skin of citrus fruits, for instance, or on the surface of the leaves, which act as the skin of the plant. This indicates the strong affinity of essential oils for the skin.

PHYSICAL PROPERTIES OF ESSENTIAL OILS

Essential oils are chemically very different from vegetable oils or other types of fats. Aromatic molecules are much smaller than fatty acids. They are carbonic chains that generally have ten carbons. A few have fifteen carbons, and some rare components have up to twenty carbons.

What characterizes essential oils is the fact that they are volatile, which means that they evaporate completely when exposed to the air. If you put one drop of vegetable oil, such as canola oil, on a piece of paper, it will stain and the stain will remain. If you put a drop of essential oil on the same piece of paper, it will eventually evaporate completely. This volatile quality is what allows us to smell essential oils in the first place. It is also the property that allows us to extract essential oils through distillation.

Essential oils are lipophilic, which means that they are readily absorbed by vegetable oils, waxes, and fats. This property allows us to make flower oils and allows the extraction process called enfleurage. The lipophilic property of essential oils is very useful for the preparation of massage oils and facial oils. It also means that essential oils applied externally absorb rapidly into the skin and the underlying tissues thanks to their high fatty content.

Essential oils are hydrophobic—that is, they do not mix with water. This property is necessary for the final stage of steam distillation, in which the essential oils are separated from the water. Hydrophobia makes essential oils difficult to use in water-based products. In general, it is not a good idea to put essential oils into water as they will float on the surface. Essential oils are partially soluble in alcohol. The amount of an essential oil that can be mixed with alcohol depends on the individual essential oil and the proof of the alcohol.

Essential oils are organic solvents. Pine oil and lemon oil, for example, are used in cleaners and polishes, orange oils in mechanical cleaners (Fast Orange), and limonene in things like Goo Gone. Turpentine, extracted from various conifers, is a paint thinner. Essential oils can dissolve styrofoam and certain plastics.

The chemistry of essential oils is rather complex. It varies during the day and throughout the year; it depends on the part of the plant being distilled (root, wood, bark, leaf, stem, flower, seed), the variety, the soil, even the climate. The oils are mainly constituted of terpenes, sesquiterpenes, esters, alcohols, phenols, aldehydes, ketones, and organic acids. They contain vitamins, hormones, antibiotics, and/or antiseptics. The yield of essential oils varies between 0.005 and 10 percent of the plant. Thus 1 pound of essential oil requires 50 pounds of eucalyptus or lavandin, 150 pounds of lavender, 500 pounds of sage, thyme, or rosemary, and 2,000 to 3,000 pounds of rose!

TRADITIONAL METHODS OF EXTRACTION

Oil Infusion and Enfleurage

Extraction by fats is probably the oldest method of extracting essential oils.

Oil infusion is an easy, do-it-yourself type of extraction. It consists of soaking any plant material—herb, flower, or seed—in vegetable oil in a glass jar and exposing it to the sun for a few days. The plants are then strained out and more herbs may be added to the scented oil. Shepherds and farmers in Provence will prepare the "red oil" by soaking St. John's wort flowers in olive oil for two weeks. This oil has amazing healing properties and is very efficient in treating burns. Oil infusions are very versatile. They can be used for culinary purposes and are also particularly well suited for making creams, ointments, liniments, massage oils, and bath oils.

In enfleurage fresh flowers are placed on top of a blend of fat (traditionally a mixture of pork fat, beef fat, and vegetable oils). The fat absorbs the aromatic oils released by the flow-

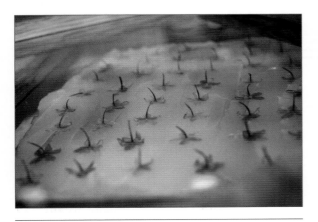

Enfleurage

ers. Every day, the old flowers are removed and fresh flowers are placed on the fat, until the right concentration of oils in the fat is reached. The oil-infused fat is called a pomade. The pomade is washed with alcohol to remove the fat, and the alcohol is removed through vacuum distillation. This process yields a form of oil called an absolute from enfleurage.

Cold Expression

Some essential oils can be extracted by cold pressure; this process is commonly used for citrus fruits. The outer layer of the fruit peel contains the oil and is removed by scrubbing. Through centrifigation, the oil then separates from the pulp. (If you pinch the peel of a lemon or an orange over a candle flame, you can see the oil come out when the peel burns in the flame.)

The Origin of Distillation

Distillation is still the most common process of extracting essential oils. Historians do not agree on its origin, but most attribute it to Avicenna, the famous Arab philosopher, physician, and alchemist who lived at the turn of the last millennium. However, Zozime, a renowned Egyptian chemist living in the third century CE, wrote about numerous designs of stills adorning the wall of a temple in Memphis. It is quite likely, in fact, that the Egyptians were aware of a primitive process of distillation.

In the first century CE, Dioscorides already wondered about the origin of distillation. He reported that, according to oral tradition, a

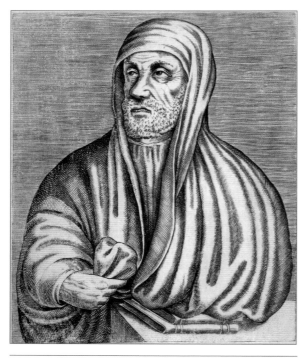

Avicenna (980–1037)

physician baked pears between two dishes. When he took off the upper dish, he noticed that the steam covering it smelled and tasted like a pear. It inspired him to build an elaborate instrument for the extraction of the "quintessences" of medicinal plants.

A still consists of a vat: a large cylindrical tank that contains the plants. Steam is sent through the plants from the bottom of the vat and evaporates the oils. The vat is covered by a special lid (*col de cygne,* or swan neck), which collects the steam and sends it to the coil, usually refrigerated with running water, where the steam is condensed. The mixture of condensed water and oil separates naturally by decantation in a *vase florentin* (florentine vase). This is illustrated in figure 3.1.

Many farms in southeastern France had such

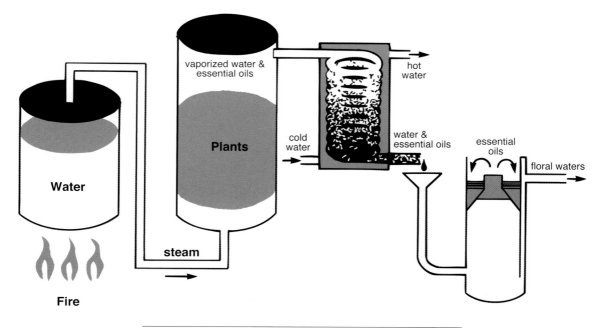

Fig. 3.1. The steam distillation process

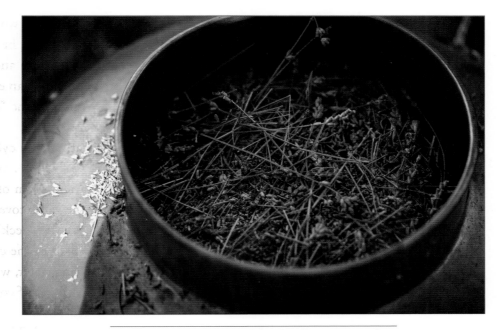

Antique copper bowl used for distillation to produce lavender essential oil

equipment until the early 1900s. Since the vats were relatively small (the main vat contained less than 100 gallons), they were often used for extracting essential oils (mostly wild lavender) in the summer and distilling brandy in the winter. Today wild lavender has almost disappeared and nobody picks it anymore (I bought one of the last batches a few years ago), but there are still many distilleries in Provence. In some areas every village has at least one. The vats are much larger (some have up to six vats containing more than 1,500 gallons), and the water is now heated in a separate boiler. The people there distill mostly lavandin, a hybrid of lavender that gives a better yield of lower-quality essential oil. They also distill true lavender, hyssop, clary sage, and occasionally tarragon or cypress.

Extraction by Solvents

This relatively modern technique is used worldwide for higher yield or to obtain products that cannot be obtained by any other process. The plants are immersed in a suitable solvent (acetone or any petroleum by-product), and the separation is performed chemically by distillation under special temperatures that condense the oil but not the solvents. Unfortunately such oils always contain some traces of solvent and are therefore not suitable for aromatherapy.

For the fabrication of "concretes," the material is usually soaked in hexane. The mixture is then concentrated by double distillation, and the final product has a creamy consistency due to the presence of residual solvents and waxes from the plants. The "absolutes" are obtained

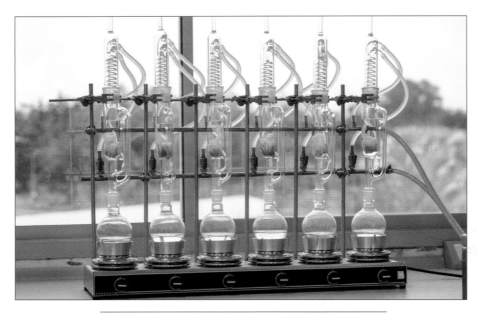

Soxhlet extractor used for extraction by solvents

from concretes by dilution in alcohol, double filtration, and double concentration, which eliminates most waxes and residual solvents.

This method is used widely for rose, neroli (orange blossoms), cassia, and tuberose. It is the only way to extract oils from jasmine, honeysuckle, carnation, and others. Concretes and absolutes are used extensively in cosmetics and perfumery; they should not be used for aromatherapy.

Supercritical Carbon Dioxide Extraction

Supercritical carbon dioxide extraction is a relatively new process that has raised great hopes among perfumers and aromatherapists. How is it supercritical?

Any substance can exist in three different states: gas, liquid, and solid. Every substance may be in any of these three states depending on its temperature and pressure. In addition, certain substances can be found in the supercritical state—that is, they are neither liquid nor gas, but rather they are both; they disperse as readily as a gas (i.e., almost instantaneously) and have solvent properties.

Under any given temperature most substances go from gaseous at low pressure (close to a vacuum for heavy substances like metal) and to liquid when the pressure increases. Some substances, though, never become liquid if their temperature is maintained over their supercritical temperature. They will instead be in the supercritical state when pressure increases over supercritical pressure.

Carbon dioxide (a fairly inert gas naturally occurring in the air that we breathe) has the power to become supercritical. Even better, its supercritical temperature is 33°C (a little more than room temperature). Supercritical carbon dioxide then becomes an excellent solvent of fragrances and aromatic substances. The advantages are that the whole operation takes place at fairly low temperature, and therefore the fragrance is not affected by heat; the extraction is almost instantaneous (a few minutes) and complete. Because the solvent is virtually inert, there are no chemical reactions between the solvent and the aromatic substances. In comparison, steam distillation requires one to forty-eight hours, it always leaves some residues of essential oils, and many substances are hydrolyzed or oxidized in the process.

Unlike the products of regular solvent extraction (concretes, absolutes, oleoresins), the solvent can be easily and totally removed just by releasing the pressure. The whole process takes place in a closed chamber, which means that even the most volatile and most fragile fractions of the fragrance can be collected. Consequently the end product is as close as anyone can get to the plant's aromatic substance.

Supercritical carbon dioxide extraction then appears to be an aromatherapist's dream come true. Unfortunately the supercritical pressure for carbon dioxide is more than 200 atmospheres (200 times the regular atmospheric pressure!), requiring very heavy and expensive stainless-steel still equipment.

Supercritical carbon dioxide extracts are now commercially available for a wide range of products such as rose, myrrh, frankincense, vanilla, cinnamon, and many spices as well as

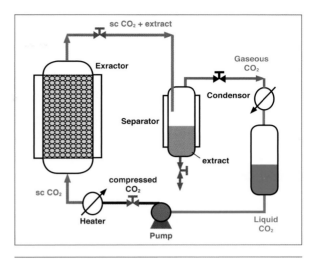

Fig. 3.2. Supercritical carbon dioxide extraction process

vegetable oils such as rosehip and pomegranate. Supercritical carbon dioxide extraction is also the most efficient method of decaffeination and is the most common method to produce CBD oil. The equipment can be ordered online from Alibaba.com.

Yield of the Most Common Essential Oils

The yield of essential oils varies greatly from one plant to another. To make 1 kilogram (kg) of essential oil, it takes about:

    20 kg of clove buds
    30 kg of eucalyptus leaves
    35 kg of lavandin
    150 kg of lavender
    300 kg of peppermint
    300 kg of Moroccan rosemary
    500 kg of red thyme
    600 kg of French rosemary

800 kg of clary sage

1,000 kg of chamomile

3,000 kg of rose

10,000 kg of melissa

The difference in yields leads to wide variations in price from one essential oil to another. Obviously eucalyptus oil will be rather inexpensive, while rose oil is going to be very costly.

Floral Waters, Distillates, and Hydrolates

Floral water, distillates, and hydrolates are obtained by sending steam through the plants and condensing this steam; they are often a by-product of distillation, in which case they are recovered from the florentine vase after separation of the essential oils. The best floral waters are obtained by cohobation, a process that continuously recycles the distillate. The amount of water used for distillation is proportional to the quantity of plant; the overflow from the florentine vase is sent back into the boiler, and steam is sent through the plant material until it is saturated.

Hydrolates contain the water-soluble active principles of the plants. They retain a small amount of essential oils (about 0.2 gram per liter), which disperses in an ionized form so that the product is less likely to cause skin irritation. Hydrolates were traditionally used for skin care, for the disinfection of wounds, and for healing. Because hydrolates are milder and easier to use than essential oils, their utility in skin care and cosmetics is considerable. Rose flower water, orange blossom water, chamomile water, and bluet water are among the most renowned.

Do It Yourself

All an amateur distiller needs is a pressure cooker. Place the plants on a screen above the water. Replace the valve with a plastic hose (2 to 5 feet long), boil the water, run cold water on the hose, and collect the floral water and oils in any suitable container. You can separate the oils by decantation in glass bottles. You will not, of course, produce large amounts of oils, but their quality will be excellent and you will also obtain plenty of floral water with which to prepare your own cosmetics, creams, and shampoos. I should warn you, however, that distillation is an incurable addiction!

HOW TO KEEP YOUR ESSENTIAL OILS

Essential oils are precious products that can be very expensive. (You will understand why when you start making your own.) Store them in tightly closed dark glass bottles to prevent their deterioration by light or by air. They should also be protected from temperature variations; prolonged heat is not good for them. Under normal conditions, essential oils can be considered fresh for three years after their extraction.

THE QUALITY ISSUE

The quality of the essential oils available on the market has improved substantially since this book's first publication, thanks mostly to better consumer education. Good-quality essential oils are now easily available through spas and skin care salons, health food stores, and specialty stores as well as direct from producers via their websites. Although some offer products with aromatherapy claims, the mass market has yet to discover real essential oils.

Quality is still an issue, and consumers should be watchful of possible adulterations, which can be natural or synthetic. There are two main reasons for adulterations. The chemical composition of essential oils of a given plant can vary to a large extent, depending on the variety, the time, the soil, and the methods of cultivation and distillation. The oil of thyme, for instance, varies from 100 percent thymol to 90 percent carvacrol, with some varieties containing citral or geraniol. In addition, many of the basic components, such as linalool, cineol, borneol, citral, and nerolidol, are present in different essences. Knowing the main components of a given essential oil, it is then possible to reconstitute it using cheaper essential oils

or their components. Rose, for instance, is often falsified with geranium, lemongrass, palmarosa, terpenic alcohol, stearine, and so forth.

Recent advances in chemistry have flooded the market with synthetic essential oils. These synthetic reconstitutions are mostly used in the food or cosmetic industry but are also used in perfumery and pharmacy. The chemical substances present in the oils are in perpetual interaction, and the kind of interaction taking place basically depends on the way these substances have been put together. The action of essential oils depends also on the processes taking place in them. Therefore natural or synthetic reconstitutions will never replace the natural oils. For aromatherapy as well as for perfumery or cosmetics, one should use only the best quality of essential oils.

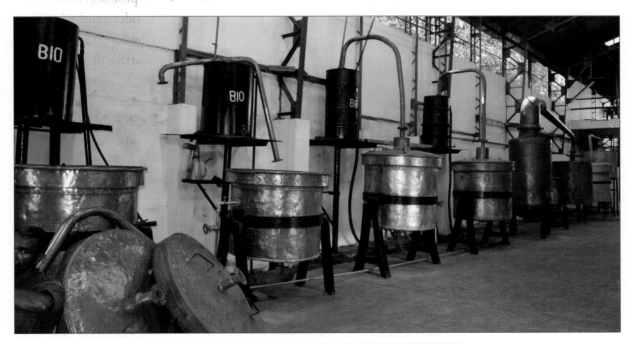

Stills used to produce ylang-ylang essential oil in
Nosy Be, Madagascar

The oils extracted by cold pressure are of course the closest to the products present in the plant, but only a few oils can be extracted by this method. Steam distillation yields the second best quality. Wild plants growing in unpolluted areas or organic plants, of course, yield the best quality of oil. Nonorganic products are not recommended, as many synthetic pesticides are soluble in the plants' aromatic substances and might be concentrated in the oil.

Various analytical processes are available for evaluating the quality of an essential oil, the most common being gas chromatography and mass spectrometry. Such methods allow an experienced specialist to detect most adulterations but will not provide any information on more subtle criteria of quality, such as country of origin or method of growth. Such methods are impractical for the average consumer who must rely on a trusted supplier.

Finding a reliable supplier is challenging because of the nature of the market: the essential oil market is rather complex, and one needs to be very familiar with it to be able to obtain optimum quality. Most of the trade in essential oils is done through brokers, and the major market for essential oils is still the fragrance and the food industries. The aromatherapy market is a growing but still marginal market. The food industry trade concerns a few selected oils, such as citrus, mint, and spices. The widest variety is being used by the fragrance industry. For that industry consistency in smell and in price is more important than purity. Most fragrance formulations include hundreds of ingredients, some natural, some synthetic. It is very important for the compounder that all ingredients maintain consistency. But nature is not consistent. From one crop to the next, from one origin to the next, the fragrance of an essential oil may vary substantially. Such variations may be buffered by addition of synthetic or natural components. Price may also fluctuate wildly. A given oil may double in price after a natural disaster in an important area of production. For instance, floods in China almost tripled the price of geranium in 1995. Price variations are buffered the same way. This explains why it can be challanging to obtain reliable quality essential oils on the open market.

Following are some guidelines for selecting a supplier of essential oils.

+ Make sure that your supplier can provide as detailed information as possible about the essential oils they offer: botanical name, country of origin, and, if possible, method of growth.
+ Price is an indication, but make sure that your supplier does not take advantage of your concern about quality to charge excessive prices: oils such as eucalyptus, especially *Eucalyptus globulus,* and orange, lemon, cedarwood, and pine are plentiful and inexpensive. Rose, jasmine, neroli, and tuberose are extremely expensive and are always sold in small amounts. Be very suspicious of such oils offered at a relatively low price.
+ Established companies with a solid reputation are more likely to have reliable sources and better buying power and therefore offer quality at competitive prices.

FOUR

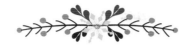

The Chemistry of Essential Oils

THE ATOMIC SAGA

Atoms consist of electrons, which have a negative electrical charge, orbiting around a nucleus. The nucleus contains the protons, which have a positive electrical charge, and the neutrons, with no electric charge. Each atom has the same number of electrons and protons, to bring the total electrical charge to zero. The electrons are disposed in layers around the nucleus. Each layer can hold a set maximum number of electrons. Thus the first layer cannot contain more than two electrons, the second layer holds a maximum of eight electrons, and so on.

Hydrogen is the most common atom in the universe and has the simplest possible structure: a single electron orbiting around one proton; it has one empty space in its single layer. Carbon, another very common atom, consists of six protons and six neutrons in the nucleus, with six orbiting electrons—two in its first layer, four in its second layer—and four empty spaces.

Oxygen has eight neutrons, eight protons, and eight electrons—two in its first layer, six in its second layer—and two empty spaces.

Atoms are impelled to fill up all their electronic layers. In fact, they compulsively need to fill up this outermost layer. If they are left alone, they usually combine with themselves. The hydrogen atoms share their electrons two by two; two oxygen atoms get together and each contribute two electrons. Carbons are a little bit different. Carbon atoms arrange themselves in three-dimensional patterns, each carbon being attached to four other carbons and contributing one electron to each liaison. Billions of billions of carbon atoms can thus be connected in huge patterns.

But most atoms seem to prefer diversity. They combine with other atoms to form molecules in a kind of atomic mating process called bonding. Atomic bonding consists of sharing the electrons in the outermost layer so as to fill up this layer. When two atoms share one electron in a molecular liaison, it is called a single bond. Atoms may also share two electrons in a double bond or even three electrons in a triple bond.

Hydrogen can form only a single bond; oxygen can form single bonds (as in water, where it is attached to two hydrogens) or double bonds (as in carbon dioxide, where two oxygens share two electrons each with a carbon). Carbon can form triple bonds, usually with itself.

By human standards atomic behavior can be rather objectionable and creepy: to fill up their outmost layer, atoms will use any possible means. They tear molecules apart to steal others' atoms, which is called an atomic reaction. And some atomic reactions can be pretty wild. Thus when you send, for instance, some oxygen atoms into a crowd of methane molecules (each made of four hydrogens attached to one carbon), the oxygen atoms are so anxious to combine that any spark causes an explosion. The oxygens split the methane; some oxygens join with hydrogens to create plain water, while others take care of the carbons in carbon dioxide. The whole exchange is brief but rather intense. This is exactly what happens when a gas leak blows up a ten-story building.

When the universe was still young and reckless, the type of atomic massacre that I just described was really nothing compared to what was going on every day. As time went by, atoms settled down in more stable molecules (burned out, probably). The interchanges became more sophisticated, especially on our planet. Molecules got bigger and bigger, until life became possible.

From general warfare, atomic behavior evolved into a harmonious dance. Under the tight control of life forces, molecules go around, gently swapping atoms or atomic groups.

Carbon is the major performer in life's molecular dance. Its blatant promiscuity and its ability to link with itself allow it to generate chains of carbon atoms. In such chains each carbon atom is linked to one (at each end of the chain) or two (inside the chain) carbon atoms. Carbons usually attach themselves to each other through a single bond. This leaves space for two or three extra bonds where hydrogen and oxygen (carbon's two major partners in life's waltz) or other radicals can be attached. Molecules as complex as DNA, life's inner memory chip, can thus be created.

The smaller molecules tend to be volatile—that is, they evaporate easily. The larger the molecule, the lower its ability to evaporate (i.e., the higher its boiling point). Essential oils are volatile; their molecules are rather small. Most of them have ten or fifteen carbon atoms (see the discussion in next section of terpenoid molecules).

THE CHEMISTRY OF COMMON ESSENTIAL OIL CONSTITUENTS*

Almost all of the molecules found in essential oils are composed of carbon and hydrogen or of carbon, hydrogen, and oxygen. The chemistry of the constituents of essential oils is determined by two factors, one artificial (the steam distillation

_____

* In collaboration with Kurt Schnaubelt, Ph.D.

process) and the other intrinsic to the plant (the biosynthesis of the constituent molecules).

By steam distillation, a process that is mainly physical, only volatile and water-insoluble constituents are isolated from the plant. The main types of chemical compounds isolated are terpenes, terpenoid compounds, and phenylpropane-derived compounds. There are many other constituents in plants (often valuable) that do not find their way into the essential oils. Among them are all the molecules that are soluble in water, like acids or sugars, or that are too large or too high in polarity to evaporate with steam, such as tannins, flavonoids, carotenoids, and polysaccharides. Three main categories of chemical compounds can therefore be distinguished in essential oils: (1) terpenes and terpenoid compounds, (2) sesquiterpenes and sesquiterpenoid compounds, and (3) phenylpropane derivatives. The first two share the same biosynthetic pathway.

Terpenes and Sesquiterpenes

Terpenes and sesquiterpenes are molecules made up of carbon and hydrogen (hydrocarbons). They provide the basic chemical structures through the ability of the carbon atom to form chemical bonds with other carbon atoms. Carbon atoms bonding to each other determine much of the overall shape and size of the molecule—they form the "carbon backbone" of the molecule. If the only other element present is hydrogen, the molecules are called unsubstituted and are referred to as terpenes or sesquiterpenes.

The terpenoid molecules share a common biosynthetic pathway. Their chemical struc-

ture can be looked at as if they were made up of multiples of the isoprene molecule. The isoprene structure consists of a chain of five carbon atoms. (Rationalizing the makeup of terpenoid molecules as multiples of isoprene units is a useful model, but the actual biosynthesis takes a different course.) The smallest molecules formed in this way are the monoterpenes, with ten carbon atoms. They are the main constituents of many essential oils.

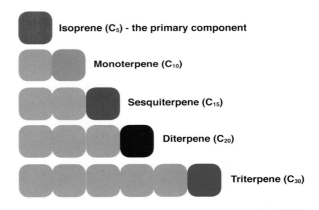

Isoprene (C_5) - the primary component

Monoterpene (C_{10})

Sesquiterpene (C_{15})

Diterpene (C_{20})

Triterpene (C_{30})

Fig. 4.1. Schematic drawing of terpenes

Molecules with fifteen carbon atoms, sesquiterpenes, are also commonly encountered in essential oils, since they are still volatile enough to distill with steam. Molecules with twenty carbons (diterpenes) are found in essential oils to a much lesser degree. Terpenoid molecules with thirty and forty carbon atoms also occur in plants but are not found in the essential oils. Their molecular weight is too high to allow for evaporation with steam. Important molecules of lifelike steroids and certain hormones are members of this last group. Monoterpenes have a ten-carbon structure, sesquiterpenes have fifteen carbons, and diterpenes have twenty carbons.

Functional Groups in Essential Oil Constituents

Unsubstituted hydrocarbons can be modified by a functional group—that is, one or two hydrogen atoms are replaced by the functional group in the molecule. Within the realm of essential oils, the functional groups we have to deal with are all formed through the different ways in which oxygen can be attached to carbon.

Generally, molecules made up of a terpene structure and a functional group are called terpenoid (or sesquiterpenoid, from sesquiterpenes). Strictly speaking, the term *terpenes* (or *sesquiterpenes*) would refer to hydrocarbons and *terpenoid* to substituted terpenes. In the professional literature, the term *terpene* (or *sesquiterpene*) is often used to denote the whole group of molecules with the same basic structure, including hydrocarbons and substituted molecules.

The properties of essential oil constituents are determined by their basic structure (mono-, sesqui-, and diterpene) and their functional group (figure 4.2).

Ketones

Thujone, pulegone, pinocamphone, and carvone are important ketones. Oxygen can be attached to a carbon through a double bond. The resulting group is called a carboxyl group; if the oxygen is attached to a carbon located within a carbonic chain, the resulting molecule is called a ketone.

Monoterpenoid ketones determine the main characteristics of a fair number of essential oils, such as hyssop and sage. Other oils with a

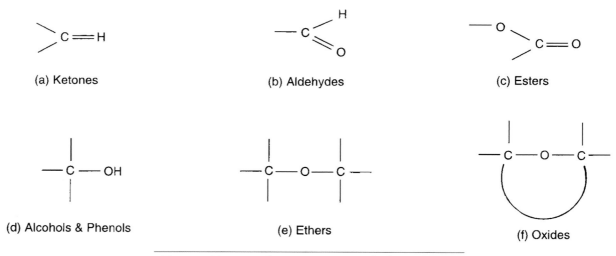

Fig. 4.2. Functional groups in essential oil constituents (C, carbon; H, hydrogen; O, oxygen)

substantial ketone content are thuja and pennyroyal (neither should ever be taken internally). The applications of these oils most relevant to aromatherapy are easing or increasing the flow of mucus and their cytophylactic effect. Both properties are utilized extensively in aromatherapy in remedies for upper respiratory complaints (mucolytic) and skin care preparations (cytophylactic). Many ketones are neurotoxic when taken internally. Some of them can be dangerous (including pulegone in pennyroyal and thujone in mugwort, *Salvia officinalis,* and thuja).

Aldehydes

Citral, citronellal, neral, and geranial are important aldehydes. Like ketones, aldehydes have a carboxyl group, but unlike ketones, their oxygen is attached to a carbon that is also linked to a hydrogen, which means that they are not located with a carbonic chain.

Monoterpenoid aldehydes are the main chemical feature of the oils of melissa (*Melissa officinalis*), lemongrass, citronella, lemon verbena (*Lippia citriodora*), and *Eucalyptus citriodora*. Studies show that aldehydes found in these oils are sedative. Citral has also been found to possess strong antiseptic properties.

Esters

Linalyl acetate, geranyl acetate, bornyl acetate, and methyl salicylate are important esters. Ester groups contain a double bond between carbon and oxygen (a carboxyl group). A second oxygen molecule is bonded to the carboxyl group,

rendering it an ester group. Esters are produced through the reaction of an alcohol and an acid. Esters are characteristically antifungal and sedative. They have a direct calming effect on the central nervous system and can be powerful spasmolytic agents.

Roman chamomile contains a number of esters that are not found commonly in other essential oils. The spasmolytic power apparently reaches a maximum in this oil.

Esters are generally fragrant and often have very fruity aromas. They are commonly used in compositions of fruit aromas and flavorings. Linalyl acetate, for instance, is found in large amounts in lavender and bergamot. It is the reaction product of linalool and acetic acid. Clary sage is another oil whose ester characteristics are obvious, especially if it is used in massage.

Esters are found in essential oils in probably larger numbers than the representatives of any of the other groups. Few essential oils have esters as the main constituent, but often even small amounts of characteristic esters are crucial to the finer notes in the fragrance of an essential oil.

Terpene Alcohols

Linalool, borneol, citronellol, geraniol, santalol, estragol, and nerol are important alcohols. Oxygen is most often attached to a terpene molecule through a single bond in the hydroxyl group, in which a hydrogen takes up the second oxygen bond. The hydroxyl group (–O–H) consists of a water molecule (H–O–H) separated from one of its hydrogen carbons, hence its name. The hydroxyl group has very strong reactive power.

Molecules with a hydroxyl group are called alcohols. They are typically very fluid. If an alcohol group is introduced into a terpene molecule, the resulting compound is called an alcohol or terpene alcohol. Terpene alcohols are among the most useful molecules in aromatherapy. The terpene alcohols found in common essential oils show a fair degree of diversity with respect to their properties as well as their fragrance, but they also have several properties in common. Terpene alcohols are generally antiseptic, and a positive energizing effect is attributed to them. Linalool is a prominent terpene alcohol in lavender, rosewood, petitgrain, neroli, and coriander. Citronellol, which has been shown to possess antiviral qualities, is a main constituent in rose and geranium oils, and geraniol is found in palmarosa. Alpha-terpineol is characteristic in *Eucalyptus radiata* and niaouli (*Melaleuca viridiflora*). Terpineol-4 is a main constituent in tea tree and garden marjoram. Other oils also in this group are present in *Ravensara aromatica* and cajeput.

All these oils have as common qualities an antiseptic nature; a pleasant, uplifting fragrance; desirable properties; and very low toxicity. The usefulness of the terpene alcohols has been pointed out again through research that suggests that those juniper oils with a high terpineol-4 content and a corresponding low content of pinenes (terpene hydrocarbons) are the safest diuretic agents among the different types of juniper oil.

Oxides

If oxygen links two carbons and at the same time is a member of a ring structure, the compound is called an oxide. Cineol, also called eucalyptole, is almost in a class of its own. As a chemical compound it is an oxide. It imparts a strong expectorant effect to the different varieties of eucalyptus oils. It is practically ubiquitous, being a more or less desired constituent of almost every other essential oil.

Linalool oxide is an important constituent of the oil of the decumbent variety of *Hyssopus officinalis*. This oil has a low ketone content and a reduced toxicity compared with the oil of *Hyssopus officinalis*.

Phenols

Thymol and carvacrol are shown in figure 4.3. When an alcohol hydroxyl group is attached to a benzene ring, the resulting compound is called a phenol. The phenol structure is strongly electropositive and therefore very active chemically. Phenols like thymol or carvacrol are the strongest antibacterial agents among the monoterpenoid compounds of aromatherapy.

Their strongly stimulant character is widely utilized in aromatherapy; however, these oils can be very irritating, and they should be used only in appropriately low concentrations.

Phenylpropane Derivatives

Eugenol, cinnamic aldehyde, anethol, methylchavicol, safrol, myristicin, and apiol are shown in figure 4.3 (also see table 1 on page 42). The common characteristic of this class of essential oil constituents is that they are all derived from

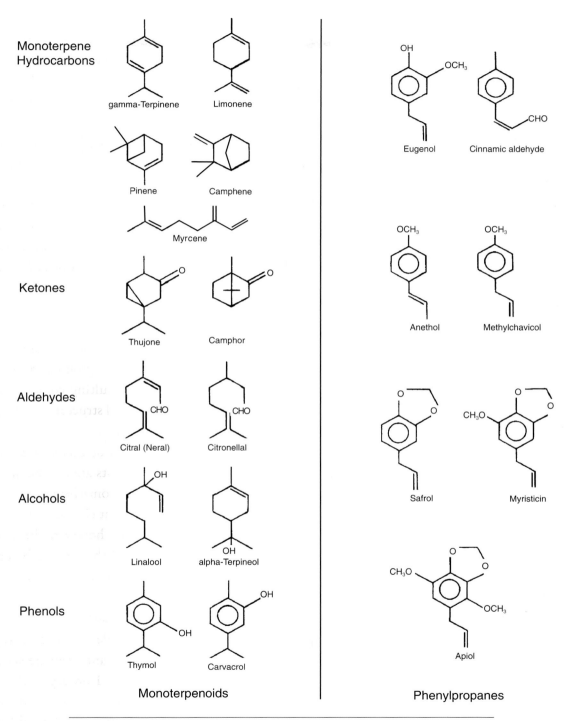

Monoterpene Hydrocarbons

gamma-Terpinene   Limonene

Pinene   Camphene

Myrcene

Ketones

Thujone   Camphor

Aldehydes

Citral (Neral)   Citronellal

Alcohols

Linalool   alpha-Terpineol

Phenols

Thymol   Carvacrol

Monoterpenoids

Eugenol   Cinnamic aldehyde

Anethol   Methylchavicol

Safrol   Myristicin

Apiol

Phenylpropanes

Fig. 4.3. Examples of Terpene and Phenylpropane Essential Oil Constituents

Table 1
Properties of Phenylpropane-Derived Essential Oil Constituents

Phenylpropane derivative	Property	Source
Eugenol	Antiseptic	Clove
Cinnamic aldehyde	Stimulant, skin irritant	Cinnamon
Anethol	Increases secretion	Aniseed
Methylchavicol	Expectorant, spasmolytic	Basil, tarragon
Safrol, myristicin, apiol	Diuretic, spasmolytic, abortive (apiol), central nervous system stimulant, hallucinogenic (myristicin)	Parsley, nutmeg, sassafras

the phenylpropane structure. The elements that make up this structure are an "aromatic" phenyl ring system with a propane (three-carbon) side chain. This basic structure of nine carbon atoms is then modified by various groups attached to it. A double bond in the side chain often allows the attached groups to interact with the pi-electron system of the aromatic ring, rendering some molecules in this group pharmacologically highly active. Their biosynthetic pathway, originating through shikimic acid, is different from those of the terpenoids.

Cinnamon and clove, like the phenolic essence, are strong antiseptic agents. They can cause severe skin reactions and must be used with caution. Eugenol, the main constituent of clove oil, in addition to being antiseptic and fungicidal, shows local anesthetic properties. It has also been reported to inhibit certain carcinogenic processes. The same effect was found for caryophyllene, another constituent of clove oil (see the

discussion of sesquiterpenes on page 45). Aniseed, basil, and tarragon are not as aggressive as cinnamon or clove can be, yet they all share a distinctly sweet character in their fragrance. The main constituents of basil and aniseed oils, methylchavicol and anethol, can cause negative effects if used in unreasonably high concentrations. Others in this group include safrol (sassafras, camphor), myristicin (nutmeg), and apiol (parsley). While most of these oils can be used beneficially in aromatherapy, they share a potential for toxicity in high concentrations or with prolonged use. The potential of nutmeg to act as a hallucinogen (dosages required to induce these effect are unsafe and can cause lasting damage or death) and the effects of anethol, well known through its abuses in anise liqueurs, demonstrate the ability of phenylpropane constituents to interact with the central nervous system in a way that depends strongly on dosage and/or concentration.

Many of the properties of terpenoid essential oil constituents (ketones, aldehydes, terpene alcohols, esters, cineol, and phenols) are listed in table 2.

Terpene Hydrocarbons

Limonene (90 percent or more of most citrus oils), pinene, camphene, and myrcene are shown in figure 4.3. With regard to their properties, terpene hydrocarbons are often thought to be rather insignificant constituents of essential oils. There has been discussion of whether terpenes are skin or mucous membrane irritants. Studies of various pine oils show that antiseptic principles are formed when these oils are subjected to natural or induced aging or oxidation. A study of the effects of terpenes against herpes simplex and other viruses should renew the respect for terpenes in aromatherapy. Limonene (the main constituent of many citrus oils), alpha-sabinene, and gamma-terpinene have all been found to possess antiviral properties. Essential oils with high proportions of monoterpene hydrocarbons include:

Lemon, orange, bergamot (limonene)
Black pepper (pinenes, camphenes, etc.)
Pine oils (pinenes)
Turpentine (pinenes, limonene)
Nutmeg (pinenes)
Mastic (pinenes)
Angelica (pinenes)

Table 3 illustrates the activities of monoterpenes as well as sesquiterpenes and diterpenes.

Table 2
Properties of Terpenoid Essential Oil Constituents

Terpenoid	Property	Source
Ketones	Promote tissue formation, mucolytic, potentially neurotoxic	Sage, thuja, wormwood (thujone), hyssop (pinocamphone)
Aldehydes	Anti-inflammatory, sedative, antiviral	Melissa, lemongrass (citrals), citronella, *Eucalyptus citriodora*
Terpene alcohols	Bactericidal, toning, diuretic, antiviral	Lavender, coriander, petitgrain, rosewood (linalool), *Eucalyptus radiata,* niaouli (alpha-terpineol), tea tree, marjoram, juniper (terpineol-4)
Esters	Spasmolytic, sedative, can be antifungal	Roman chamomile (angelica acid esters), lavender, clary sage, bergamot (linalyl acetate)
Cineol	Expectorant	Eucalyptus and many other oils
Phenols	Bactericidal, immunostimulant, stimulant, skin irritant, potentially toxic to liver	Thyme (thymol), oregano, savory (carvacrol)

Table 3
General Effects of Terpenoid Compounds*

Activity	Monoterpenes	Sesquiterpenes	Diterpenes
Anesthetic	+		
Analeptic	+	+	
Analgesic		+	
Anthelmintic	+	+	
Antiarrythmic		+	
Antibiotic (antibacterial, antifungal, antiseptic, antiviral)	+	+	+
Antiepileptic		+	
Antihistaminic	+		
Anti-inflammatory, antiphlogistic	+	+	
Antirheumatic	+		
Antitumor (antiblastic, anticarcinogenic, cytotoxic)	+	+	+
Choleretic, cholagogue		+	
Diuretic	+		
Expectorant	+		+
Hypotensive	+	+	+
Insecticidal	+		+
Irritant	+	+	
Juvenile hormone		+	
Pheromone	+	+	
Phytohormone (growth regulating)		+	+
Purgative	+		+
Sedative	+	+	
Spasmolytic	+	+	
Toxic		+	+
Vitamin			+

*The biological, pharmacological, and therapeutic activity of normal monoterpenes (and also of many sesquiterpenes) is closely connected to that of the essential oils. An overview of the most important biological properties of mono-, sesqui-, and diterpenes is given here.

Sesquiterpenes

Chamazulene, bisabolol, santalol, zingiberol, carotol, caryophyllene, and farnesol are among the important sesquiterpenes. Table 4 lists some sources of sesquiterpenes.

As we look at sesquiterpene constituents of essential oils, the influence of a functional group becomes less dominating. The increased size of the overall structure brings about increased complexity. The interaction between carbon backbone and functional group becomes more subtle and intricate. The individuality of the molecule becomes a greater factor in the makeup of the pharmacological effect of the molecule.

More than two thousand sesquiterpenes have been isolated from plants to date, and their structures vary widely. Most of these sesquiterpenes can be attributed to thirty main structural types. A summary of their biological activity is shown in table 5. Essential oils with a high proportion of sesquiterpene constituents are mostly distilled from roots and woods or from plants of the Asteraceae family.

Sesquiterpenes have been the object of much interest and research into their properties. The bulk of that research has been performed on sesquiterpenes isolated from plants of the Asteraceae family that are not common essential oil plants. The situation for the aromatherapist is somewhat unsatisfactory, since there are good reasons to speculate on the potential properties of sesquiterpenes in essential oils but only limited availability of substantiating research data. There are some notable exceptions. In the effort to provide a scientific basis for the many uses of German chamomile (*Chamomilla matricaria*), the antiphlogistic properties of chamazulene and alpha-bisabolol were firmly established.

Table 4
Sources of Sesquiterpenes in Essential Oils

Sesquiterpene	Property	Source
		From roots
Zingiberol		Ginger
Vetiveron, vetiverol	Stomachic, carminative	Vetiver
Complex composition (almost 100% sesquiterpenes)		Spikenard
Valeranon (valepotriates C 101)	Sedative, spasmolytic	Valerian
		From woods, seeds, or leaves
Alpha-santalol		Sandalwood
Patchouli alcohol		Patchouli
Carotol		Carrot seed
Nerolidol (dependent on type)	Disinfectant, antiseptic	Niaouli
		From the plant family Asteraceae
Chamazulene, bisabolol	Antiphlogistic	German chamomile
Chamazulene (dependent on chemotype)		Yarrow, tansy

Table 5
Sesquiterpenes from Essential Oils with
Known Pharmacological Properties

Sesquiterpene	*Property*	*Source*
Chamazulene	Antiphlogistic, anti-inflammatory	German chamomile, yarrow, tansy
Caryophyllene	Sedative, antiviral, potentially anticarcinogenic	Clove (10%); occurs in many essential oils in low concentrations
Farnesol	Bacteriostatic	Rose, chamomile, and many other flower oils

Farnesol is a sesquiterpene whose superior properties as a bacteriostatic and dermatophilic agent are well documented. Because of its ability to inhibit, rather than kill, the growth of bacteria, it is an ideal deodorizing agent, since it inhibits the development of odor-causing microorganisms without eliminating the bacteria that are present on healthy skin.

Finally, caryophyllene, which is found in many essential oils, most notably in clove oil, has received renewed attention. It combines sedative and antiviral effects with an ability to inhibit some carcinogenic processes.

Sandalwood illustrates the lack of solid research data on sesquiterpenes that are found in essential oils. On one hand, there is ample anecdotal evidence for its usefulness in urinary tract infections, and even pharmacological textbooks list it as a potential urine disinfectant. On the other hand, an antibacterial effect of sandalwood oil constituents has not been confirmed. It is of course tempting to speculate that searching for an outright bactericidal effect of santalol may be the wrong experiment in light of the fact that sesquiterpenes can be effective immune stimulants. The effect of the oil could be caused not through direct bactericidal action but rather through stimulation of the body's defense mechanisms.

A summary of essential oils and their major chemical components is given in table 6.

Chemotypes

Certain plants and other organisms categorized under the same species, subspecies, or varieties with identical morphological characteristics display substantial variations in the chemical composition of some of their organic compounds, such as alkaloids and essential oils. Such variations are called chemotypes and are probably related to minor genetic and epigenetic variations or may be caused by climatic and other environmental conditions.

Chemotypes are widespread within the botanical family of Lamiaceae in plants such as basil, lavender, melissa, oregano, peppermint, rosemary, sage, and thyme. Geranium is another plant with many chemotypes.

Table 6
Essential Oils and Their Major Chemical Components

Plant	Number of carbons	Components
Angelica	10	Musk ketone
Aniseed	9	Phenylpropane (*trans*-anethole)
Basil	9	Phenylpropane (methylchavicol)
Bay	10	Phenylpropanes: myrcene, eugenol, chavicol
Bergamot	10	Terpenes and esters: limonene, linalyl acetate
Birch	8	Esters: methyl salicylate
Cajeput	10	Terpene alcohols: alpha-terpineol
Caraway	10	Ketones: limonene, carvone
Cardamom	10	Terpenes: cineol
Carrot seed	15	Sesquiterpene alcohol: carotol
Cedarwood	15	Ketone: atlantone-7
Chamomile, blue	14	Sesquiterpenoids: chamazulene
Chamomile, German	15	Sesquiterpenoids: bisabolol, chamazulene
Chamomile, mixta	10	Alcohol: ormenol
Chamomile, Roman	9	Esters
Champaca, *Michelia alba*	10	Terpene alcohol
Cinnamon bark	9	Phenylpropane: cinnamic aldehyde
Cinnamon leaf	9	Phenylpropane: eugenol
Cistus	15	Terpenes, sesquiterpenes, diterpenes
Citronella	10	Aldehydes: citronellal
Clary sage	15	Esters: linalyl acetate, sesquiterpene alcohol
Clove buds	9	Phenylpropane-phenol, eugenol
Coriander seeds	10	Terpene alcohols: linalool
Cumin seeds	10	Aldehyde: cuminaldehyde
Cypress	10	Terpenes: terpenyl acetate
Elemi	10	Terpenes: limonene, elemol
Eucalyptus australiana	10	Cineol
Eucalyptus citriodora	10	Aldehydes: citronellal
Eucalyptus globulus	10	Cineol, *t*-alcohol
Everlasting	15	Esters: neryl esters
Fennel	10	Phenylpropane: *trans*-anethole
Fir	10	Terpenes
Frankincense	10	Terpenes: phellandrene, camphene, olibanol

Table 6 *(continued)*
Essential Oils and Their Major Chemical Components

Plant	*Number of carbons*	*Components*
Geranium	10	Alcohols: citronellol, geraniol
Gingerroot	15	Sesquiterpenoids: zingiberone
Grapefruit	10	Terpenes: limonene
Hyssop	10	Ketone: pinocarvone
Jasmine	9	Benzyl acetate, jasmone
Juniper	10	Terpenes, terpene alcohol
Laurel	10	Cineol
Lavender	10	Esters, terpene alcohols: linalyl acetate
Lavandin	10	Esters, terpene alcohols: linalool, camphor, linalyl acetate
Lemon	10	Terpenes, aldehyde: limonene, citral
Lemongrass	10	Aldehyde: citral
Lime	10	Terpenes, aldehyde: limonene, citral
Litsea cubeba	10	Aldehyde: citral
Lovage root	10	Lactones
Marjoram	10	Terpene alcohols: terpinen-4-ol
Marjoram, wild Spanish	10	Phenol
Melissa	10	Aldehyde: citral
Mugwort	10	Ketone: thujone
Myrrh	10	Terpenes
Myrtle	10	Terpenes, terpene alcohols
Neroli	10	Terpene alcohols, esters: linalool, geraniol, nerol
Niaouli	10	Terpenes, terpene alcohols
Nutmeg	9	Terpenes, alcohols: linalool, borneol, myristicin
Orange	10	Terpenes
Oregano	10	Phenol: carvacrol
Palmarosa	10	Terpene alcohols: geraniol
Patchouli	15	Sesquiterpenoids: patchoulol
Pennyroyal	10	Ketone: pulegone, methone
Pepper	10	Terpenes: piperine
Peppermint	10	Terpene alcohols: menthol, carvone, linalool
Petitgrain biguarade	10	Terpenes, esters: linalyl acetate
Pine	10	Terpenes

Table 6 *(continued)*
Essential Oils and Their Major Chemical Components

Plant	Number of carbons	Components
Rose	10	Alcohols: citronellol, geraniol, nerol
Rosemary	10	Terpenes, terpene alcohols: cineol
Rosewood	10	Terpene alcohols: linalool
Sage, Spanish	10	Cineol, camphor, esters
Sandalwood, Mysore	15	Sesquiterpenoids: santalol
Savory	10	Phenol: carvacrol
Spearmint	10	Terpene alcohols: carvone
Spike	10	Terpene alcohols: linalool, camphor
Spikenard	15	Sesquiterpene alcohol
Spruce	10	Terpenes
Tangerine	10	Terpenes
Tarragon	9	Phenylpropane: methylchavicol
Tea tree	10	Terpenes, terpene alcohols: terpinen-4-ol
Therebentine	10	Terpenes: p-menthadienes
Thyme, citriodora	10	Aldehyde: citral
Thyme, lemon	10	Alcohol: linalool
Thyme, red	10	Phenol: thymol
Verbena, lemon	10	Aldehyde: citral
Vetiver	15	Sesquiterpenoids: vetiveron, vetiverol
Ylang-ylang	10	Alcohols: geraniol, linalool, ylangol

FIVE

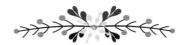

Principles of Aromatherapy

How Essential Oils Work

Aromatherapy is rather different from other healing modalities in that it acts on various levels, each in synergy with the other levels. Aromatherapy treats symptoms by addressing the specific physical, energetic, and psychological background of the individual client.

BIOPHYSICAL ACTION OF ESSENTIAL OILS

Essential oils have measurable biophysical actions when inhaled, ingested, or applied to the body. There are some general properties that we find to a greater or a lesser degree in all essential oils due to the fact that essential oils are made primarily of terpenoid compounds. However, each individual essential oil has specific properties due to its specific chemical composition.

Healers and pharmacists have long made use of essential oils' biophysical actions. Essential oils have been used in pharmaceutical preparations since the beginning of pharmacy in Egypt more than six thousand years ago and are still used in Europe, Asia, and the United States. In France, cough preparations, digestive aids, muscle liniments, and wound preparations found in virtually every pharmacy contain essential oils as active ingredients. In the United States, Vicks VapoRub includes peppermint, eucalyptus, and several other essential oils as active ingredients. Originating from Asia, the world-famous Tiger Balm is made primarily of essential oils.

Medicinal Properties Found in Most Essential Oils

Antiseptic Property

A property universally found in essential oils is the antiseptic property. All essential oils are antiseptic to some degree. The most antiseptic are the oils with a high phenolic content. Phenolic compounds found in essential oils are thymol, carvacrol, and eugenol. These compounds are found in especially large quantities in red thyme, savory, oregano, clove, and cinnamon. Such oils are extremely powerful antiseptics, but they should be used with caution because they can be irritating, especially when applied to the skin. Phenol-rich essential oils should be used only under medical supervision.

In addition to the very aggressive phenolic oils, aromatherapy provides us with a wide choice of milder but very effective essential oils for antiseptic use. These include all the oils rich in alcohols, such as geranium, all the various lavenders, palmarosa, tea tree, marjoram, and ylang-ylang. These oils are much milder than the phenol-rich oils and are very safe to use. They are useful for home remedies and first-aid kits, and they work well on minor wounds, as prevention from infectious diseases, and for skin care.

Oils rich in terpenes include pine and most members of the Coniferae family (fir, spruce, cedarwood, juniper) and the citruses (lemon, lime, orange, grapefruit, tangerine). These oils are slightly more aggressive than the alcohol-rich oils but are still very safe to use. They are especially efficient when used in a diffuser.

Expectorant

In addition to their overall antiseptic properties, most essential oils are expectorants to some degree, which means that they stimulate the fluidification and expulsion of mucus from the lungs. As we know, the lungs produce mucus to filter the air that we breathe. Mucus traps the dust and pollutants that we breathe all day long. It is very important that we expel mucus properly, especially when we live in polluted cities. Essential oils are helpful for this purpose.

The most effective expectorant oils are those that are rich in a chemical called cineol

and include most members of the Myrtaceae (eucalyptus, myrtle, niaouli, cajeput) and the Coniferae (pine, spruce, fir, cedarwood) families. *Eucalyptus globulus* is one of the most powerful expectorants.

Cytophilactic

Most essential oils are cytophilactic, which means that they stimulate cellular activity and cellular regeneration. The most cytophilactic oils are geranium, lavender, rosemary, sandalwood, and, generally, all the oils rich in alcohol.

Rubefacient

Essential oils are rubefacient, which means that they activate capillary circulation. This is especially true of oils rich in phenols (thyme, oregano, savory, clove) and, to a lesser degree, oils rich in oxides (eucalyptus, niaouli, cajeput, rosemary) and terpenes (pine, fir, juniper).

MAJOR MEDICINAL PROPERTIES OF INDIVIDUAL ESSENTIAL OILS

Each essential oil also has specific properties, depending on its chemical composition. The major medicinal properties found in some essential oils are listed in table 7 on page 52.

ACTION OF ESSENTIAL OILS ON THE SKIN

Essential oils are extremely beneficial for the skin. In fact, the use of essential oils in skin care can be traced back to the Egyptians, the inventors of cosmetology. The Egyptians had extremely elaborate skin care regimens, which could take hours to complete. Their skin

Table 7
Medicinal Properties of Individual Essential Oils

Property	Essential oils
Sedative/calming	Neroli, spikenard, lavender, chamomile, marjoram, ylang-ylang
Energizing/stimulant	Peppermint, ginger, nutmeg, pepper, rosemary, lemon, eucalyptus, pine
Antispasmodic (cramps, colics, PMS, cough)	Cypress, Roman chamomile, tarragon, lavender
Anti-inflammatory	Blue and Roman chamomile, helichrysum
Emmenagogue (regulates female hormonal system)	German chamomile, clary sage, fennel, mugwort, lavender
Aphrodisiac	Jasmine, champaca flowers, ylang-ylang, clary sage, sandalwood, patchouli, cistus, pepper
Analgesic/pain killer	Clove, birch, red thyme, rosemary

care preparations made extensive use of aromatic substances.

The skin is a barrier between our bodies and the outside world. Thus the skin absorbs and filters elements from the air and absorbs a small amount of air (the skin breathes). It also absorbs moisture and other elements applied to the skin. The skin must filter germs and unwanted substances such as pollutants. This double function of the skin is extremely important. At the same time, our bodies expel moisture to help control body temperature. The skin expels sebum, a waxy substance that our bodies use as a protectant; it also expels various waste materials through the sebaceous glands.

Essential oils help the skin perform its role as a barrier. This is a very important property for skin care. In addition, some of the basic properties of essential oils make them extremely useful for skin care.

ACTION OF ESSENTIAL OILS ON THE ENERGETIC LEVEL

Essential oils are considered the life force, the energy, of the plant. They are used with great efficiency in energy work such as acupressure, Shiatsu, and chakra work. Specific essential oils can be associated with each meridian and chakra. See tables 8, 9, and 10.

ACTION OF ESSENTIAL OILS ON THE EMOTIONAL LEVEL

Essential oils are first and foremost fragrances, and as such they have deep effects on the emotional plane. Table 11 on page 56 describes which essential oils to use to influence specific moods.

Table 8
Action of Essential Oils on the Skin

Property	Essential oils	Special applications
Antiseptic	Tea tree, eucalyptus, niaouli, lavender, geranium	Cleansing, protecting and treating acne-prone skin*
Cytophilactic/cellular stimulant	Myrrh, frankincense, rose, sandalwood, geranium, rosemary, lavender	Treatment and healing of minor skin lesions and blemishes, mature skin
Rubefacient	Juniper, grapefruit, rosemary, red thyme (in very small doses)	Toxin elimination, lymphatic drainage, treatment of sluggish conditions
Astringent	Geranium, lemongrass, lemon	Skin toner, treatment of oily skin
Regulator	Sage	Sebaceous secretions, treatment of oily skin
Protectant	Palmarosa, sandalwood, myrrh	Protect skin, help it retain moisture
Soother	Chamomile, neroli, rosewood, rose, ylang-ylang	Sensitive skin, couperose, broken capillaries

*Caution: Do not use oregano or clove on skin; use red thyme only in very low concentration on skin.

Table 9
Essential Oils and Meridians
(Refer to Fig. 5.1, Meridian charts, on page 54)

Meridian	Essential oils
Lungs	Myrtaceae family (*Eucalyptus globulus, australiana,* and *smithii;* myrtle; niaouli; cajeput), Coniferae family (fir, pine, spruce, cedarwood, cypress), hyssop, lavender
Liver	Sage, rosemary, lemon, peppermint, chamomile
Stomach	Umbelliferae family (aniseed, angelica, fennel, caraway, coriander, tarragon), ginger, orange, peppermint, chamomile
Intestine	Savory cinnamon (bark and leaf), ginger, angelica, tarragon, fennel, caraway, coriander, cardamom

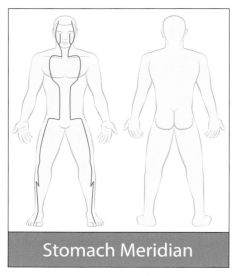

Stomach Meridian

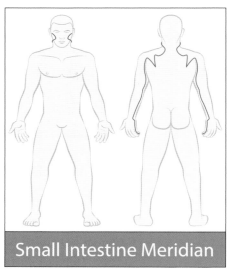

Small Intestine Meridian

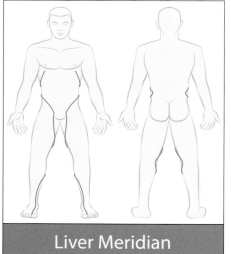

Liver Meridian

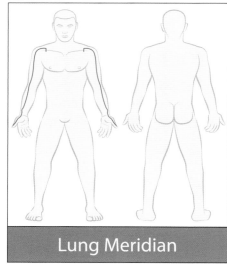

Lung Meridian

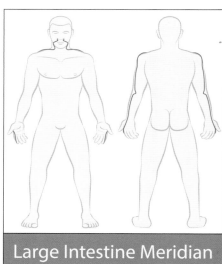

Large Intestine Meridian

Fig. 5.1. Meridian charts

Table 10
Essential Oils and Chakras
(Refer to Fig. 5.2, Chakra chart)

Chakra	Essential oils
Root	Vetiver, spikenard, angelica, ginger, cedarwood, spruce
Sacral	Jasmine, champaca flowers, ylang-ylang, pepper, clary sage, patchouli, sandalwood
Solar plexus	Rosemary, ginger, nutmeg, sage, pepper, thyme
Heart	Neroli, rose, marjoram, melissa
Throat	Geranium, eucalyptus
Third eye	Mugwort, sandalwood, cedarwood, vetiver
Crown	Cistus, rose, jasmine, sandalwood, spikenard

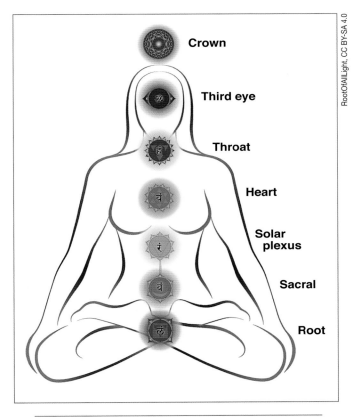

RootOfAllLight, CC BY-SA 4.0

Fig. 5.2. Chakra chart

Table 11
Action of Essential Oils on the Emotional Level

Mood	*Essential oils*
Gratifying/indulging/ warming/loving	Jasmine, ylang-ylang, rose, neroli, sandalwood, absolutes of tuberose, mimosa, narcissus, champaca flowers
Vitality/stimulating	Rosemary, juniper, peppermint, basil, Coniferae family, Myrtaceae family
Balancing/calming/ soothing	Lavender, marjoram, chamomile, neroli, ylang-ylang, tangerine, melissa, spikenard
Mental concentration, centering/deepening	Bursearaceae family (myrrh, frankincense, elemi), sandalwood, cistus, spruce, Coniferae family
Clarifying/sharpening (for confusion)	Petitgrain, peppermint, basil, rosemary, Myrtaceae family
Memory stimulation	Juniper, basil, rosemary
Emotional shock, grief	Rose, neroli, marjoram, clary sage, chamomile
Stress	Chamomile, neroli, marjoram, lavender, ylang-ylang
Sadness	Benzoin, jasmine, rose, clary sage
Dream work	Mugwort, clary sage, cistus
Psychic work	Cistus, sandalwood, spikenard, rose
To build confidence, self-esteem	Alternate between gratifying oils in the evening and vitality oils in the morning (see first two table entries above)

ACTION OF ESSENTIAL OILS ON THE SPIRITUAL PLANE

Aromatic substances have been used for ritualistic purposes since the origins of human culture. It was, in fact, one of their first uses. Traditional cultures viewed fragrances as a link between the human realm and the gods. Fragrances in most ancient cultures were considered a gift from the gods. The shamans or priests used them to carry their offerings to the kingdom of the gods. Even to this day, all major religions, whether Shintoism, Buddhism, Hinduism, Islam, or Christianity, use incenses and scented oils in their rituals and ceremonies.

Essential oils, especially the oils from woods and gums, have a very centering and opening effect on the psyche. They help create a sense of connectedness, community, and elevation, and they inspire the sacred in each of us. The major oils for ritualistic purposes are sandalwood, cistus, myrrh, frankincense, benzoin, vetiver, spikenard, and rose.

When Mary Magdalene wanted to express her devotion to Christ, she washed his feet with the famous nard oil (now known as spikenard), one of the most expensive oils of antiquity, brought by caravans from the Himalayas to Palestine. She incidentally spent a fortune on

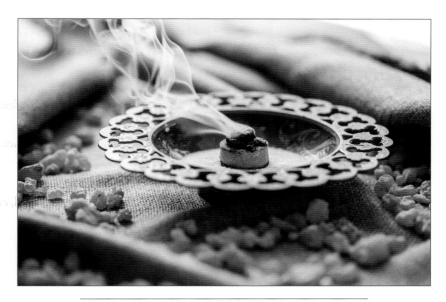

Frankincense burning on a hot coal

Christ's feet, provoking the anger of Judas, the bookkeeper of the group.

This episode from the Bible inspired a blend that I created more than ten years ago, when a French religious group asked me to create a Good Friday blend to reenact the foot washing. I later added this blend to my Aroma Véra line under the name Sacred Synergy; it's now discontinued. It combines the major ritualistic oils of all major spiritual traditions.

CONCLUSION

The various levels of action of essential oils are not exclusive from one another. On the contrary, whatever the application, we always encounter the various effects to one degree or another. When doing skin care or body care treatments in particular, there will be not only physical effects and effects on the skin but also effects on the energetic level and on the emotional level. Each level of action works in synergy with the others to enhance the overall effect.

The capacity to affect people on so many different levels—physical/medicinal, skin, energy, emotional/psychological—is really what makes aromatherapy so special. No other healing art has such versatility and broadness of action.

This capacity is also what makes aromatherapy such a creative art. The possibilities are endless; one can go as far as he or she wishes. Aromatherapy offers unique opportunities to fine-tune and personalize treatments to an extreme degree. The trained technician can design treatments that take into account the client's biophysical background, skin type, energy level, and emotional and psychological states. Mastering aromatherapy is a challenging but uniquely rewarding venture.

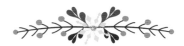

SIX

Comparative Study of Modes of Administration

Benefits, Risks, Applications, and Contraindications

Aromatherapy is an art and a science, but it is not a cult or a religion. It cannot solve all the problems of the planet and it does not work miracles, but it can play a role in dedicating ourselves to living closer to nature, and it can help relieve many common (and some not-so-common) conditions.

This chapter will review the various routes of administration of essential oils (olfactory, pulmonary, transdermal, and internal), including their benefits, risks, applications, and contraindications. We also will discuss the most common misunderstanding regarding the internal use of essential oils.

Essential oils have many different levels of action: biophysical, energetic, emotional, mental, and spiritual. We will review how each route of administration is best suited to each level of action, and we will see how aromatherapists can best design their treatment to optimize the

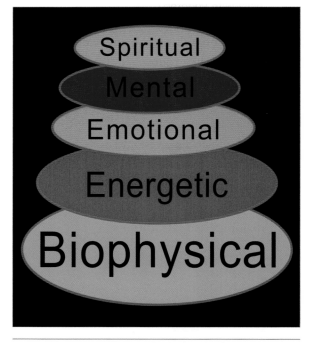

Fig. 6.1. Essential oils' levels of action

effects of essential oils by using the best mode of administration for the intended effect.

Brief Reminders

It is very important to understand what essential oils are so that they can be used efficiently and safely. Before we start going over the various modes of administration and their risks and benefits, let's quickly review some basics.

- Essential oils are chemically very different from vegetable oils and other types of fats. The aromatic molecules are much smaller than the fatty acids and are readily absorbed through the skin.
- Essential oils are volatile—they evaporate completely when exposed to air.
- Essential oils are lipophilic—they mix very easily with vegetable oils and fats.
- Essential oils are hydrophobic—they do not mix with water.
- Essential oils are partially soluble in alcohol.
- Essential oils are organic solvents.

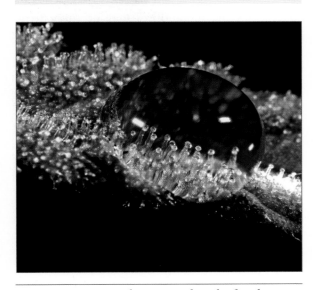

Secretory trichomes on plant leaf with water drop for size comparison

BODY BARRIERS AND ADMINISTRATION

Our body is protected from noninvasive exposure to unwanted substances and pathogens by three physical barriers: the skin, the digestive tract, and the respiratory system. The brain is further protected by an internal barrier, the blood-brain barrier. Contrary to common belief, the skin is not our largest protective barrier. The surface area of the digestive tract, if all its folds, nooks, and crannies were unfolded, is more than 350 square meters. As for the lungs, with three hundred million or so alveoli, the total surface area is around 70 square meters. The skin, in comparison, is only about 2 square meters.

These barriers also provide the routes of entry for the substances that our body depends on for its survival—the air we breathe, the liquids we drink, the food we eat—as well as other substances, such as drugs, be they pharmaceutical or recreational, and pollutants. We rely on these same routes for the noninvasive administration of substances via inhalation, ingestion, and transdermal application. Injection is the major invasive route of administration.

Our body's natural barriers are our interface with our environment. They work in symbiosis with the microbiota, the aggregate of microorganisms that resides on or within a number of human tissues and biofluids, to process any substances with which we come in contact.

After administration by one of these routes, substances go through the following stages:

+ Absorption
+ Distribution
+ Storage
+ Metabolism
+ Excretion (urine or feces)

Absorption

Absorption is the process by which the administered substance crosses the barriers to enter the body and reach the bloodstream through lymphatic circulation and the capillaries. The amount absorbed and the rate of absorption depend on the substance and the route of administration.

Distribution

Distribution is the movement of substances throughout the body through the circulatory system. Certain substances may be attracted to specific organs or systems, either by design for therapeutic purposes or with adverse toxic effects in the case of pollutants.

Storage

Certain substances may be stored in various parts of the body, such as fat or bone, to remain there for anywhere from a few days to years or decades. For example, marijuana stays in the body for one to three months, depending on body fat content; opiates stay for three to seven days; cocaine and methamphetamines stay for three to five days; alcohol stays for twelve to twenty-four hours; and nicotine stays for one to ten days. Pesticides like DDT (which is currently banned in most of the world) can stay in the human body for years or even decades. Lead is stored in the bones for decades, and asbestos stays in the lungs forever. Essential oils may stay in the body for a few hours to a few days, depending on the oil.

Metabolism

Most substances absorbed into the body interact with various endogenous chemicals secreted by organs such as the stomach, intestines, pancreas, and liver and are thus transformed, in a process called metabolism, into new substances called metabolites. For example, when macronutrients—carbohydrates, proteins, fats—are metabolized, their breakdown provides the body with the energy to run cellular processes and forms the building blocks for proteins, lipids, and nucleic acids.

Metabolism tends to produce substances that are easier for the body to excrete, but in some cases the metabolites may be more toxic than the original substance that was absorbed. Ingested tetrahydrocannabinol (THC) is metabolized into 11-hydroxy-THC, which is much more psychoactive than THC and takes much longer to cross the blood-brain barrier. The liver turns alcohol into acetaldehyde, which is far more toxic and damaging than alcohol itself. Acetaldehyde is usually turned rapidly into acetic acid (our harmless, good old vinegar), but this second conversion lags with heavy drinking, causing headaches, nausea, palpitations, and flushing. Carriers of a genetic mutation prevalent among some populations of Asian origin—Han Chinese, Taiwanese, Japanese, and Korean—

have no acetaldehyde-metabolizing capacity and are almost completely alcohol intolerant.

Excretion

When the absorbed substances and their metabolites have accomplished their function, the leftovers and by-products are excreted as body waste. The kidneys eliminate water-soluble waste as urine. The large intestine eliminates solid waste as feces. The lungs eliminate carbon dioxide. Volatile substances such as alcohol are also partially released through the lungs. The lungs also trap dust and pollutants with their cilia and mucus, which are then excreted in the mucus.

BIOAVAILABILITY

Whether we are talking about administering nutrients, nutraceuticals, or pharmaceuticals or being exposed to toxins, pathogens, or pollutants, an important factor to consider is bioavailability, broadly defined as the proportion of substance that is absorbed and distributed in the body. Bioavailability varies a lot depending on the route of administration, the physicochemical properties of the substance, and the physiology of the user.

Bioavailability is 100 percent for injected substances, but it varies from 0 to 100 percent for inhaled substances and topical applications, and it varies substantially for ingested substances, too, as we will see in the next section. Bioavailability decreases with time unless the substance or its metabolites are stored, in which case bioavailability may remain relatively

constant for long periods of time, usually with adverse consequences.

THE BLOOD-BRAIN BARRIER

The brain is further protected by the blood-brain barrier (BBB), a highly selective semipermeable border that separates the circulating blood from the brain and extracellular fluid in the central nervous system and prevents the free flow of substances from systemic circulation to the brain or cerebrospinal fluid.

Water, carbon dioxide, oxygen, and lipid-soluble molecules are able to move freely across the BBB by passive diffusion. Molecules such as glucose and amino acids that are crucial to neural function are selectively transported across it. However, the BBB blocks bacteria and large or hydrophilic molecules.

Essential oils, being made of small lipophilic molecules, can cross the BBB. In some cases that can be risky; essential oils containing thujone, for example, are neurotoxic and can be dangerous, especially to people subject to seizure.

ROUTES OF ADMINISTRATION OF SUBSTANCES

The main routes of administration of substances —whether drugs, food, or others—are the

+ respiratory system (nasal cavity and lungs),
+ mucous membranes (nasal, sublingual, vaginal, and anal),
+ skin (transdermal administration),
+ digestive system (oral administration), and
+ injection.

The Respiratory System

Administration of substances via the respiratory system targets the nasal cavity and the lungs, both of which allow fast absorption into the bloodstream. It also targets the olfactory system within the nasal cavity, which transmits olfactory stimuli but is not normally considered an absorption channel.

The Olfactory Pathway: Scent Stimulation

The olfactory pathway is a sensory system. It transmits stimuli, not substances, and therefore is not a mode of administration per se. However, as we shall see below, some substances, such as psychoactive substances, may be absorbed directly into the brain through a process known as olfactory transfer.

The olfactory mucosa is a specialized part of the respiratory mucosa that lines the upper region of the nasal cavity. It consists of the olfactory epithelium covered by a thin layer of connective tissue, the lamina propria. The olfactory epithelium contains the bipolar olfactory receptor neurons and basal cells, which are stem cells that continuously regenerate olfactory receptor neurons and supporting cells.

The olfactory system and the hippocampus are the only parts of the brain that have been observed to undergo continuing neurogenesis (the production of neurons by stem cells) in adult mammals. In the olfactory system this neurogenesis takes place in the olfactory bulbs as well as outside the brain, in the olfactory epithelium, which is replaced every six to eight weeks.

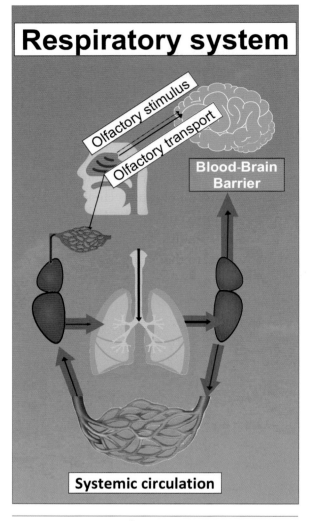

Fig. 6.2. The respiratory system

Glial cells called olfactory ensheathing cells are found in the olfactory epithelium, the olfactory nerve, and the olfactory bulbs. They ensheath the nonmyelinated axons of olfactory receptor neurons and assist the growth and regeneration of olfactory axons. Olfactory ensheathing cells have gotten scientists quite excited thanks to their axonal regeneration property. These cells have been successfully harvested and used in clinical trials to study their potential in spinal cord repair and the treatment of neurodegenerative diseases such as Parkinson's and Alzheimer's diseases.

When we smell something, what's happening is that odorant molecules, such as aromatic molecules, stimulate the olfactory receptor neurons. Even very small amounts of odorant substances can cause an olfactory stimulation. The receptor neurons transmit information about the olfactory stimulus to the olfactory bulbs and, from there, to the thalamus and the amygdala, which is part of the limbic system.

The limbic system is involved in the perception of emotions, which may explain why scents can generate strong emotions. The effects of olfactory stimulation are mostly subconscious and become conscious only when we are exposed to new olfactory stimuli.

The olfactory pathway is the ideal channel for emotional and spiritual effects. The olfactory bulbs are like an extension of the brain, and they are directly connected to the olfactory epithelium and the mucosa. The olfactory mucosa is the only part of the body where neurons are exposed directly to the external environment.

Olfactory (Transcribrial) Transfer

The fact that the olfactory system provides direct access to the brain raises an intriguing question: Can certain substances be absorbed through the olfactory mucosa and into the olfactory bulb, bypassing the blood-brain barrier?

One limiting factor for the olfactory transfer of substance is the small surface area of the olfactory epithelium, at just 10 square centimeters, which limits the amount of substance that could be absorbed. Also limiting is the location of the olfactory epithelium at the very top of the nasal cavity. The nasal cavity has a total surface area of 150 square centimeters, consisting mostly of respiratory epithelium. Several experiments suggest that olfactory transfer is achievable but may not be sufficient to reach therapeutic level.

Olfactory transfer is probably a factor in the effects of snorted psychoactive substances such as cocaine or heroin; the olfactory transfer may provide an instant effect while the effect of nasal absorption is delayed by five minutes or more. Experiments on rodents demonstrate the transfer of morphine along the olfactory pathway to the central nervous system after nasal administration.

Currently, olfactory transfer is being investigated as a route to deliver stem cells to the central nervous system in cases of neurodegenerative

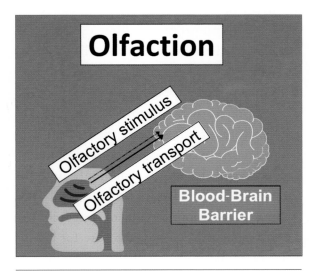

Fig. 6.3. Olfactory transfer

diseases. But the process is still poorly understood, and it is not clear whether hydrophobic substances, such as essential oils, can use this delivery pathway to the brain.

Nasal Cavity: Nasal Absorption

Nasal absorption has long been used as a method of administration in medicine as well as for recreational drug use and is ideal for substances that are active in low doses, such as essential oils.

The nasal cavity is covered by a thin, well-vascularized mucosa, allowing the transfer of substances across the epithelial cell layer and directly into the systemic blood circulation.

Nasal administration is convenient, noninvasive, and an easy method for self-administration. When a substance is sniffed or sprayed into the nose, absorption may take as little as five minutes for smaller molecules, with a bioavailability of close to 100 percent, nearly duplicating the effects of injection without its inconvenience.

Nasal administration is limited by the volume that can be administered into the nasal cavity and subject to a high variability in the amount of drug absorbed. Upper airway infections and irritation of the nasal mucosa may increase the variability. Repeated use raises the risk of harmful long-term effects on the nasal epithelium.

Intranasal delivery is commonly used for anesthetics and analgesics, steroids, and anti-asthma medication. A lot of research has recently gone into its potential use for a wide range of applications ranging from vaccines to hormones, peptides, and insulin.

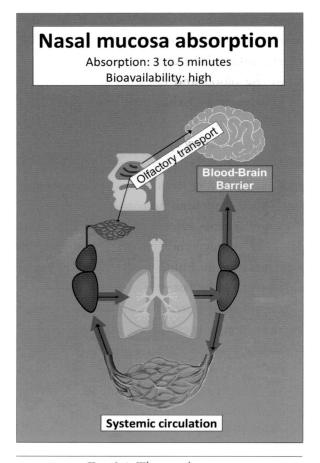

Fig. 6.4. The nasal mucosa

Upon inhalation, either with a diffuser or an inhaler, some essential oils can be absorbed via the nasal cavity.

The Lungs

The lungs have a fractal structure with a total surface area of around 70 square meters, allowing rapid and efficient oxygenation of the blood. Upon inhalation, air flows through numerous passageways, called bronchi and bronchioles, to approximately three hundred million alveoli. Alveoli are the tiny airspaces where gaseous exchange with the capillaries takes place; carbon dioxide is removed from the blood and oxygen is absorbed into the bloodstream. Exhalation expels the carbon dioxide–laden air.

The respiratory system is the most efficient and fastest route of administration for many substances, including macromolecules, with rapid absorption and high bioavailability, both for local and systemic effects. Substances that can be absorbed through the lung tissue quickly reach the bloodstream. Pulmonary administration, as it's known, is the fastest and most potent delivery route for psychoactive substances, which, by definition, can cross the blood-brain barrier. This explains why psychoactive substances such as crack cocaine, crystal meth, heroin, and opioids are far more addictive when smoked than even when injected.

Small lipophilic molecules, such as essential oils, are absorbed within seconds after inhalation, while small hydrophilic molecules need a little more time, being absorbed within up to about ten minutes.

Most of the substances that cannot be absorbed by the lungs are subsequently expelled through the mucus, but some substances, such as coal powder, tar from smoke (from tobacco or other sources), asbestos, and other pollutants, tend to accumulate in the lung tissues and cause long-term damage, such as cancer and degenerative diseases.

Essential oils, being volatile aromatic compounds, have a natural affinity for the respira-

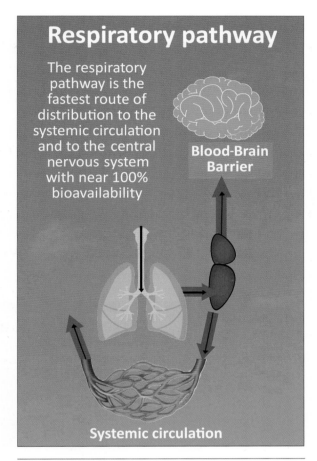

Fig. 6.5. The respiratory pathway

tory system. Nebulization is the most efficient method of pulmonary administration. One drop is approximately 0.05 milliliter, with a diameter of approximately 5 millimeters and a total contact surface area of 0.65 square centimeter. The same drop broken by nebulization into droplets of 5 microns in diameter has a total contact surface area of 650 square centimeters—a thousand times more.

Administration by respiratory routes is thus the most efficient method to use essential oils and provokes effects at all levels: physical, energetic, emotional, and spiritual.

Mucous Membranes

Mucosal absorption includes the route of nasal absorption, discussed earlier, as well as sublingual (under the tongue) absorption, vaginal absorption, and anal absorption. It is a relatively fast absorption method yielding high bioavailability, but its uses are limited by the high sensitivity of mucous membranes. Many substances may cause irritation, as is the case with phenolic essential oils such as thyme, oregano, and clove.

The Skin: Transdermal Administration

The skin is our tightest barrier. Substances applied to the skin must penetrate the stratum corneum, the outermost layer of the epidermis, which is primarily composed of ceramides, cholesterol, and fatty acids. Substances that pass through the stratum corneum must then penetrate the dermis, the hypodermis, and adjacent tissues before they can enter the bloodstream through lymphatic circulation and the capillaries.

Repeated exposure of the skin to irritating substances may cause dermatitis. That damage

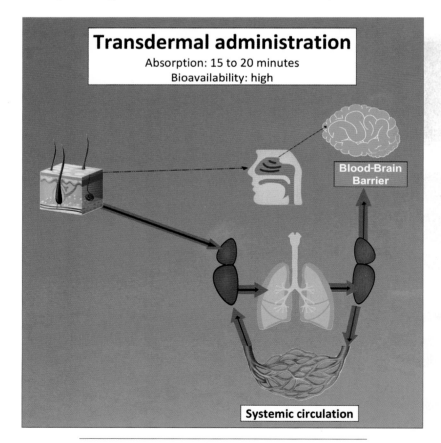

Fig. 6.6. Transdermal administration

reduces the skin's ability to serve as a barrier. Pathogens may be absorbed through skin irritations such as lesions, wounds, or even mosquito bites.

Transdermal application is made through a wide range of products, including oils, creams, foams, gels, lotions, ointments, and transdermal patches. The transdermal route is ideal for local effects and, of course, for skin care. Because essential oils are small molecules and highly liposoluble, they can quickly penetrate the dermis and epidermis. Substances that can be absorbed through the transdermal route offer a very high level of bioavailability. Transdermal administration allows for the design of very fine and precise treatments, targeting specific organs and functions, with effects on all levels: physical, energetic, emotional, and spiritual.

The Digestive System: Oral Administration

The digestive system consists of the digestive tract and accessory organs (the teeth, tongue, salivary glands, liver, gallbladder, and pancreas).

The digestive tract (gastrointestinal tract) is a continuous tube with two openings: the mouth

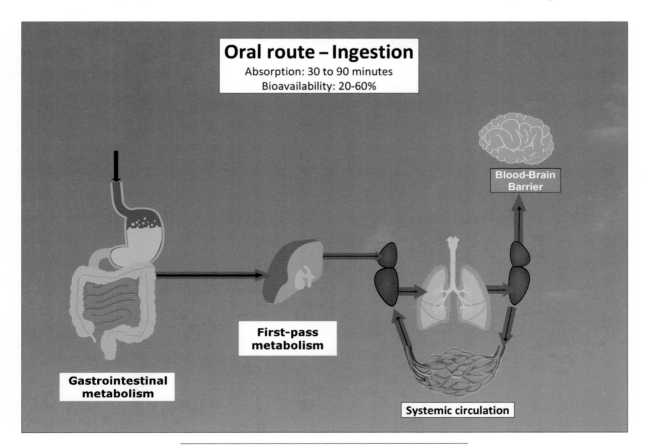

Fig. 6.7. Oral administration

and the rectum. Substances that pass through the digestive tract do not technically enter the body until they are metabolized and absorbed through the walls of the digestive tract. From the digestive tract, they can go to the liver or the lymphatic system and then on to the bloodstream.

Digestion is the mechanical and chemical breakdown of food into small molecules that are then absorbed into the body. While the other routes of administering substances are rather selective and do not transform those substances in any meaningful way, the digestive system can absorb a wide range of substances—liquids, solids, and everything in between—and transform them into chemicals that barely resemble what was ingested. In a sense, the digestive system is the body's chemical factory.

The chemical breakdown is done by the enzymes and the intestinal flora—that is, the complex community of microorganisms (bacteria, fungi, protozoa, and yeasts), sometimes called probiotics, that live in the digestive tract. The intestinal flora not only help the body break down and digest food but also are responsible for the synthesis of some vitamins and nutrients. For example, normal intestinal flora help the body create vitamin K. They also aid mineral absorption and help transform certain types of starches and sugars into energy sources for the body.

The balance of our intestinal flora system is relatively fragile and can be affected by various drugs, especially antibiotics and antiseptics. Essential oils, being antiseptic and bactericidal, can also affect the intestinal flora.

Drugs administered orally are first broken down and may be chemically destroyed or altered in the stomach, and from there they are further metabolized in the intestines. Any metabolites and remaining drug residues that are absorbed through the intestinal walls are transported through the portal vein to the liver, where they undergo a process called first-pass metabolism. The phenomenon (also known as the first-pass effect or presystemic metabolism) is is the process by which the concentration of a drug is considerably reduced before it reaches the systemic circulation. Among its other functions, the liever detoxifies the body of potentially harmful chemicals, breaking them down and processing them for excretion. When the liver receives drugs or their metabolites from the bloodstream, it works in this manner to deactivate them. Consequently their first pass through the liver greatly reduces their bioavailability. The greater the efficiency of the first step, the lesser the volume of the drug and its metabolites that reaches systemic circulation in the body.

Substances absorbed through the digestive system take a relatively long time to reach the blood because they are subject to metabolism within both the digestive system and the liver before they can reach the bloodstream. While the bioavailability of macronutrients—carbohydrates, fats, protein—is usually quite high, at more than 90 percent, the bioavailability of micronutrients (vitamins and minerals) as well as bioactive phytochemicals can vary widely. The bioavailability of lipophilic substances, such as essential oils, can be greatly improved by using lipids—oils or other fats—as carriers.

Internal use is generally the slowest, most wasteful, most inefficient, and most potentially harmful way to use essential oils. It loses all the subtle effects linked to olfaction. It is, however, the best way to treat any condition related to the digestive system and can be powerful in treating certain conditions such as infectious diseases. But the internal use of essential oils is controversial, in large part due to regulatory reasons. Many aromatherapists fear that internal use and related therapeutic claims may prompt regulators to classify essential oils as pharmaceutical drugs, with potentially catastrophic consequences for the aromatherapy industry.

While many, myself included, warn against the potential dangers of the internal use of essential oils, the fatalities that can be attributed to essential oils over the past fifty years can probably still be counted on two hands. Meanwhile, Johns Hopkins University researchers estimate that medical errors cause about 251,000 deaths per year in the United States, making it the third leading cause of death in the country.

Injection

Injection, whether intravenous, intramuscular, subcutaneous, or intradermal, is the most common invasive route of substance administration. The bioavailability of injected substances is 100 percent, and the onset of action ranges from fifteen to thirty seconds for intravenous,

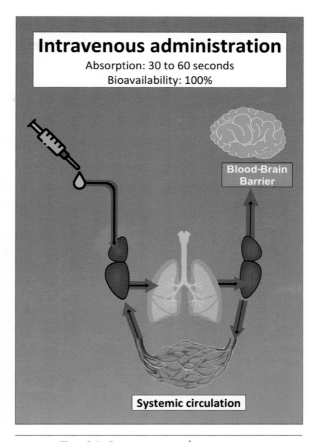

Fig. 6.8. Intravenous administration

ten to twenty minutes for intramuscular and intradermal, and fifteen to thirty minutes for subcutaneous.

Injection is particularly well suited for drugs that are poorly absorbed or ineffective when taken orally, or whenever fast effect is desirable, such as in the event of an emergency. Intravenous infusions can be used to deliver continuous medication or fluids.

Among the disadvantages of injection are need for trained staff and a sterile environment, potential pain or discomfort for the patient, an increased risk of side effects and even overdose if the dose has been calculated incorrectly, and a risk of infection from contaminated needles.

It should be noted that mosquito bites are by far the most common invasive mode of administration, delivering unwanted viruses and bacteria to unsuspecting victims. Mosquitoes claim more than three million lives worldwide every year,

making the pesky little buggers the living beings most lethal to humans, being even more lethal than human themselves. Meanwhile, human-to-human violence causes more than 1.6 million deaths worldwide, the vast majority by firearms, making them the second most lethal invasive substance delivery method.

Injection is not a method of administration used with essential oils.

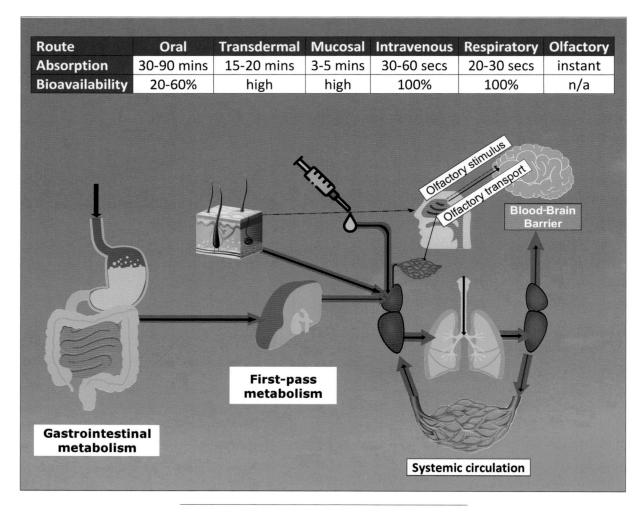

Route	Oral	Transdermal	Mucosal	Intravenous	Respiratory	Olfactory
Absorption	30-90 mins	15-20 mins	3-5 mins	30-60 secs	20-30 secs	instant
Bioavailability	20-60%	high	high	100%	100%	n/a

Fig. 6.9. Route of administration

Table 12
Routes of Administration of Substances

Route of administration	Time until action takes effect	Bioavailability	Comments
Olfactory	Instant	Does not apply	Transfers aromatic stimuli, not substances
Inhalation	20–30 seconds	100%	Ideal for essential oils
Intravenously	30–60 seconds	100%	Does not apply to essential oils
Mucous membranes/ sublingual	3–5 minutes	High	Few drugs can be absorbed in this way
Intramuscular route	10–20 minutes	100%	Does not apply to essential oils
Rectal route	5–30 minutes	50%	Reduces the effect of first-pass metabolism; inconvenient for many people
Transdermal/topical	15–20 minutes	Up to 90%	Very user-friendly; allows precise targeting of specific organs or functions
Oral route/ingestion	30–90 minutes	Low to medium	Slow and inefficient; first-pass metabolism can significantly reduce bioavailability

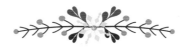

SEVEN

The Use of Essential Oils for Health, Beauty, and Well-Being

Essential oils are pleasant and easy to use. They can be used in many different ways; however, particular methods are more suited to particular applications. For instance, the diffuser is the best way to treat lung conditions, while massage is the best application for muscle pain or rheumatism. The various methods of application of essential oils can be used in conjunction. Massage, bath, and diffuser, for instance, work wonders when used in combination.

The major methods of using essential oils are

+ *internally* (by ingestion, though essential oils should be taken internally only under direct supervision of a physician),
+ *through inhalation,*
+ *through the skin* (massage, bath, friction, application),
+ *skin care and cosmetic use* (facial, compresses, masks, lotions, creams), and
+ *hair care.*

Whether taken internally or externally, essential oils diffuse through the skin and membranes and penetrate deeply into the tissues and the circulatory system. Therefore external application is a very efficient way to treat specific organs. As a rule, ingestion is indicated only for infectious diseases and to act on the digestive system (throat, stomach, liver, etc.). A massage of the corresponding zone is very helpful in such cases. In any case, essential oils should be taken internally only under supervision of a trained specialist.

INTERNAL USE

Some adepts of aromatherapy tend to glamorize internal use. They wrongly feel that they have been initiated or have graduated to some higher level of aromatherapy when they start using essential oils internally. They are reinforced in that attitude by unscrupulous marketers who market their oils as "pharmaceutical grade" or "therapeutic grade" fit for internal use, intended for the rarefied few who have been initiated in the internal art. These marketers usually charge a stiff premium for their products. In fact there are no recognized standards for pharmaceutical-grade or therapeutic-grade essential oils. To be suitable for internal use, or for aromatherapeutic use in general, essential oils should be pure, natural, and preferably derived from wild or organic plant material.

Internal use of essential oils is not safe and is not even very efficient unless they are taken in capsules or time-release form. When taken through the mouth in drops, the essential oils are mostly absorbed by the tissues in the mouth. Whatever reaches the stomach can provoke heartburn and is very hard on the liver. In fact, regular internal use of essential oils can severely damage the liver. Most of the essential oil will be destroyed in the digestive tract and will never make it to the bloodstream. In the end, internal use is usually a harmful and inefficient method of application. The few reported accidents and all of the handful of fatalities from use of essential oils involved internal use.

It is true that in some cases internal use can be very efficient: two drops of peppermint oil on the tongue will quickly clear upset stomach, nausea, or motion sickness; two or three drops of rosemary on a piece of brown sugar will get rid of a hangover after a wild party. Roman chamomile clears sluggish digestion or minor food poisoning. Fennel will promote lactation in nursing mothers. Likewise, cinnamon or savory in capsules are great for intestinal infections. But in most cases, internal use of essential oils concerns medical practice and is generally not advised self-medication.

Essential oils can be taken undiluted on a small piece of sugar or mixed with honey. In this case it is very important to carefully respect the doses. Any oil can be dangerous at high doses; the most toxic are, in decreasing order, rue, pennyroyal, thuja, *Lavandula stoechas,* mugwort, nutmeg, *Salvia officinalis,* hyssop, anise, and fennel. These oils should *never* be taken internally under any circumstances. As a rule, when other essential oils are taken internally, the maximum dose should be five drops three times a day.

For internal use, do not dilute pure essential oils in a cup of hot or cold water. Hot water will evaporate most of the essential oil; with cold water, most of the essential oil will stick to the walls of the cup. Do not use disposable plastic or styrofoam cups because essential oils, being solvents, will dissolve them and you will end up ingesting dissolved plastic.

For a more flexible and convenient option for internal use, you can dilute essential oils in ethyl alcohol (such as rum or vodka). Mix ¼ ounce of essential oils (either a single oil or a blend) in 4 ounces of 90 percent ethyl alcohol (do not use rubbing alcohol). This will give you a 6 percent preparation (for preparations in metric, use 6 milliliters of essential oil in 100 milliliters of alcohol). Take fifteen drops up to three times a day. The maximum dose is sixty drops a day.

The most efficient and safer way to use essential oils internally is to blend them in a carrier oil, such as sweet almond, coconut, or borage, at a 20 percent concentration, or fifty drops in 8 milliliters of carrier oil. Take ten drops up to three times a day, preferably in enteric capsules for release in the intestine. The maximum dose is fifty drops a day.

Aromatic Honey

Mix ¼ ounce of your blend of essential oils in 16 ounces of honey for a 2 percent preparation (2 milliliters of essential oil or blend of oils in 100 milliliters of honey).

Stir thoroughly.

Dose: ½ teaspoon three times a day.

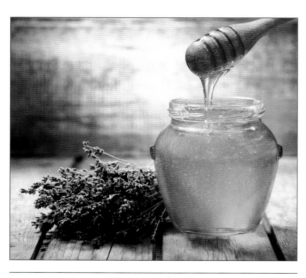

Aromatic honey

Absorption, Distribution, and Bioavailability

Ingested essential oils are absorbed and distributed within thirty to ninety minutes, with a bioavailability of 20 to 50 percent depending on various factors such as food intake and how the essential oils are ingested; optimum bioavailability is achieved by mixing essential oils with a carrier oil in an enteric capsule for intestinal release.

Ingested essential oils act mostly at the biophysical level.

Contraindications

Children, pregnant women, and people subject to heartburn or ulcers should not use essential oils internally.

The essential oils that are rich in ketones (thuja, pennyroyal, mugwort, hyssop, *Salvia officinalis, Lavandula stoechas*) should *never* be used internally. When ingested, ketones can provoke seizure or coma and can be fatal at rather low dosages.

APPLICATION OF ESSENTIAL OILS THROUGH THE OLFACTORY AND RESPIRATORY SYSTEMS

The use of aromatic fumigations is probably as old as humanity. Priests, sorcerers, and healers of all traditions used them extensively in their ceremonies and various rituals. Ancient Egyptians burned perfumes in the streets and inside the temples. More than two thousand years ago, Hippocrates, the father of Western medicine, successfully struggled against the epidemic of plague in Athens by using aromatic fumigations throughout the city. In the Middle Ages people burned pine or other fragrant woods in the streets in times of epidemic to cast out devils. Perfumers were known to resist disease.

The application of essential oils through the olfactory and respiratory systems is the easiest, most pleasant, and, in most cases, most effective way to apply them. This method requires minimal patient action: all the patient has to do is turn on a proper diffusing device, which disperses essential oils into the air, and breathe! This application method is the best and easiest way to introduce a newcomer to the world of aromatherapy.

Various devices have been designed to disperse essential oils into the air. Essential oils can be diffused in a mist with an atomizing diffuser, vaporized through heat in a candle diffuser or scented candle, or dispersed using a room spray.

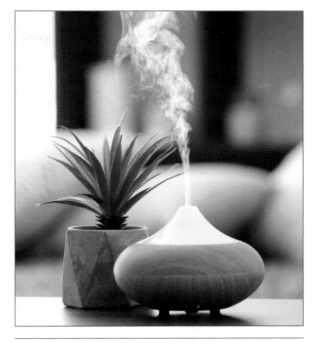

Atomizing diffuser

Inhalation Devices

Nasal inhalers generally consist of a small plastic or metal container with a cotton wick that can be soaked in essential oils. Steam inhalers vaporize essential oils for respiratory distribution and provide the added benefit of steam, which loosens mucus. Inhalation provides almost instantaneous absorption with very high bioavailability.

Cold Diffusion

The Atomizing Diffuser

The atomizing diffuser is the most effective way to disperse essential oils into the air. It is recommended for all diseases related to the lungs, the heart, the brain, and the blood. The atomizing diffuser projects drops of essential oils into a nebulizer, using air as a propellant.

The nebulizer acts as an expansion chamber in which the drops of oil are broken into a very thin mist. This mist, consisting of tiny, ionized droplets of essential oils, remains suspended for several hours, revitalizing the air with the antiseptic and deodorant properties of the essential oils. The oxidation of the essential oils provokes the formation of low doses of natural ozone that decomposes in ionic nascent oxygen. This process, occurring naturally in forests, has an invigorating and purifying effect. The atomizing diffuser is particularly effective since it diffuses the oils without altering or heating them. Since air is the propellant, there is no chemical pollution.

Through the atomizing diffuser, we experience all the various levels of action of essential oils at their maximum efficiency. It can be used for almost all prescriptions of aromatherapy. It is the subtlest, easiest, and most pleasant way to apply essential oils. It can be installed in any public or private place where air treatment is needed: saunas, hot tubs, hospitals, consulting rooms, waiting rooms, gymnastic centers, schools, and, of course, at home, in the living room, bedroom, kitchen, or bath.

A lot of clinical research on the use of this apparatus demonstrates the biophysical action of essential oils applied through diffusion. In addition to the antiseptic action, already widely documented, there is a very strong action on the lungs and the respiratory system in general (asthma, bronchitis, cold, sinusitis, sore throats, etc.). The effect on the circulatory system, the heart, and the nervous system is also very pronounced.

The lungs are one of the main energy centers. Proper breathing allows for a better energy level. The absorption of essential oils through the respiratory system is one of the best ways to activate them on the energy level. There is an obvious connection between the psychic centers and the lungs. Most spiritual practices emphasize the importance of breathing. Breathing essential oils diffused through an atomizing diffuser can thus be seen as the best way to experience the subtle effects of essential oils on the emotions, the spirit, and the soul.

Sprays

Essential oils can be dispersed into the air through a room spray. This method has the advantage of being extremely easy and portable.

It can be used in many places where a diffuser is not practical (bathroom, car, garbage can, etc.). However, it creates fairly large droplets, which limit its efficiency, and, of course, this method only diffuses for a fraction of a second.

Heat Diffusion

Essential oils can also be dispersed into the air through a heat source, in which case they are vaporized. This method is not as efficient as cold diffusion, which creates a mist, especially for therapeutic purposes.

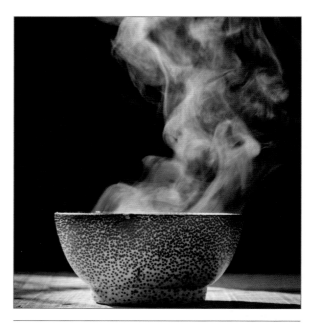

Heat diffusion

Candle Diffusers

In the candle diffuser, a small candle (votive or tea light) is placed underneath a well that holds the oils. The heat vaporizes and disperses the oils.

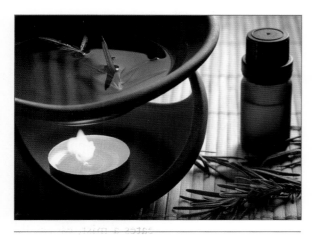
Candle diffuser

Aromatic Candles

Aromatic candles contain 5 to 8 percent essential oils in their wax. When the wax melts, the essential oil is released. This is the most inefficient way to diffuse essential oils because a large percentage of the oils are burned by the flame.

Dosage

The use of essential oil in a diffuser is generally very safe provided that you use your common sense. For an average size room the recommended use is fifteen to thirty minutes, two or three times a day. Permanent use can be appropriate in an open space, such as a store, or in large spaces, such as a large office, a spa, or a large house with open floor plan.

Some Oils to Use in Diffusion

The sense of smell is very subjective; you might particularly like some fragrances and dislike others, depending on so many factors that it is impossible to tell which one will be your favorite. In addition, your appreciation will depend on your mood, the time of the day, the season, and so on.

Calming (evening): Lavender, marjoram, chamomile, tangerine

Stimulant (morning): Sage, rosemary, pine, mints

Aphrodisiac: Ylang-ylang, jasmine, champaca flowers, sandalwood, patchouli, ginger, peppermint, pepper, savory

Lungs: Eucalyptus, lavender, pine, cajeput, copaiba, hyssop

Nervousness: Mugwort, petitgrain, marjoram, neroli

Hypertension: Ylang-ylang, lavender, lemon, marjoram

Hypotension: Hyssop, sage, thyme, rosemary

Antidepressants: Frankincense, myrrh, cedarwood

Purifier: Lavandin, lemongrass, lemon, pine, chamomile, geranium, oregano

Revivifier: Pine, fir, black spruce

Brain strengthener and memory fortifier: Basil, juniper, rosemary

Insomnia: Neroli, spikenard, marjoram, chamomile

See appendices 1 and 2 for more specific indications.

Absorption, Distribution, and Bioavailability

Respiratory administration offers the fastest absorption and highest bioavailability of all the administration methods, but much depends on the specific method. With candles and heat diffusers, for example, the quantities of essential oils actually administered can be extremely small or almost negligible for all except olfactory effects. Nasal or steam inhalation provide the highest levels of actual administration, as most of the essential oil that is released is absorbed in the respiratory tract.

Inhaled essential oils act on all levels: biophysical, energetic, emotional, mental, and spiritual.

Caution and Contraindication

Use the diffuser with extreme caution around people subject to allergies, emphysema, or asthma, and around newborn babies. In such cases use the diffuser for only a few minutes at a time. If any adverse reaction occurs, discontinue immediately. Do not use oils rich in ketones (thuja, pennyroyal, mugwort, hyssop, *Salvia officinalis, Lavandula stoechas*) in a diffuser.

BODY CARE USES OF ESSENTIAL OILS

Massage

Essential oils are particularly beneficial in massage, a slow, diffuse, gentle, and pleasant way to apply them. They are completely absorbed by the skin in 60 to 120 minutes and penetrate deeply into the tissues. Their prolonged action amplifies the effects of the massage itself. Hand healing and massage are probably the most ancient healing arts, and oils, usually scented, have been part of the treatment since its beginning.

Massage goes much further than a mere tissue manipulation. It is a direct and simple form of communication between the massage therapist and patient, where the hands are extremely sensitive receptors. During the course of the massage, the hands will discover the internal geography of the body, unraveling tensions, sores, hidden pains, sensitive points, congested areas, and swollen parts, and they will tell a lot about the patient. This is why, to give the full benefit of a massage, the massage therapist must be in an open, understanding, and compassionate state of mind.

In massage the hands are channels of healing energy; they heal at the physical, emotional, and psychic levels. Therefore aromatherapy massage is an excellent therapeutic combination as essential oils and massage have mutually enhancing effects. The massage itself will help the oils penetrate into the tissues and direct them to where they are needed most, while the essential oils will treat locally or via the energy channels (nerves and meridians). You can use massage oils after the bath to moisturize and soften the skin. You can, of course, use different oils for different parts of the body, especially if you want to act on different organs.

How to Prepare a Massage Oil

Always use ultrafiltered cold-pressed or expeller-pressed oils as a base for your massage oil. If you use cold-pressed oils, it is important that the oils that you use have been ultrafiltered. Regular cold-pressed oils contain a certain amount of organic residues that will manifest as cloudiness or deposits at the bottom of the bottle. Such

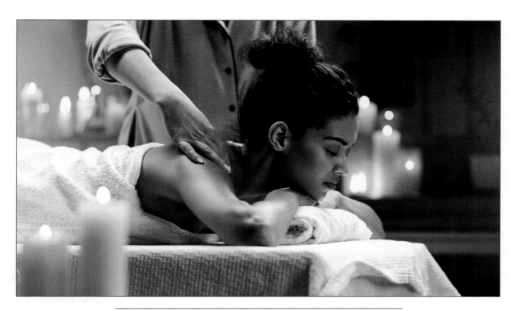

Massage

residues add to the richness and flavor of the oil for cooking but are undesirable for massage as they may cause pore clogging.

Sweet almond oil is most commonly used, but it becomes rancid very easily. Grapeseed and canola oils are fine oils with a good shelf life; they easily absorb while providing a good slip and are widely used by massage therapists and beauticians. Hazelnut oil is very rich and nourishing, although rather expensive. Peanut oil and coconut or palm oils are too heavy and may cause skin breakout. A small amount of vitamin E oil will bring some vitamins to your skin and act as a natural antioxidant.

I recommend the following oils as a blend for a massage oil base (4-ounce preparation).

Canola oil: 2 ounces
Grapeseed oil: 1.5 ounces
Wheat germ oil: 0.5 ounce

The essential oil concentration for a massage oil depends on the type of massage and the application; see tables 13 and 14 (pages 80 and 81).

Note that partial massage is massage of only one part of the body (such as shoulder massage or massage of the hips) or massage of a particular organ (stomach, liver, lungs, etc.). Topical uses are applications on a very small area such as pressure points, chakras, energy points, or meridians. Acute conditions requiring this type of application are those such as rheumatism, arthritis, or tense, painful muscles.

Caution

✦ Do not use deep tissue massage on varicose or spiderweb veins. Use only gentle, light massage.

✦ Do not use oils rich in ketones (thuja,

Table 13
Dosage for Massage Oil

Type of massage	Recommended dose			Maximum dose		
	%	Drops/100 ml	ml/100 ml	%	Drops/100 ml	ml/100 ml
Full-body massage	1.5	50	1.5	4	120	4
Partial massage	3	100	3	6	200	6
Topical use, acute conditions	6	200	6	10	333	10

pennyroyal, mugwort, *Salvia officinalis, Lavandula stoechas*), especially on pregnant women.

✦ Use only very low concentrations of phenolic oils (cinnamon bark and leaf, clove, oregano, savory, red thyme).

✦ In general, it is recommended that you decrease the essential oil concentration when working on pregnant women.

✦ Always use low concentrations on young children (cut dosages in half).

✦ Do not use essential oils in massage on people undergoing chemotherapy without proper medical supervision.

Aromatic Baths

From Egypt to India, the ancients had elaborate ritual ablutions that were combinations of hot and cold baths, ointments, and aromatic massages. Essential oils and baths have synergistic effects. Essential oils enhance the pleasure of the bath, and to quote Robert Tisserand, "If they please the nose, they also please the spirit. Then there is the physiological action of the essences on the nervous system and the rest of the body" (*Aromatherapy to Heal and Tend the Body,* 1989).

Dosage for Aromatic Baths

Aromatic baths are generally very safe provided that the essential oils are properly dispersed into

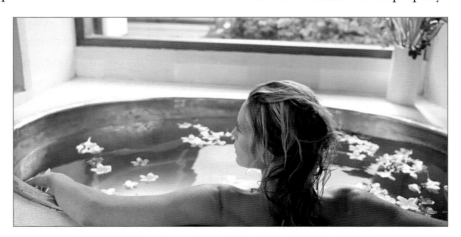

Aromatic bath

the water. Essential oils do not mix with water. Therefore it is always recommended to use a dispersant whenever using essential oils in a bath.

You can use an unscented liquid soap or foaming bath gel, a base for bath oil (we recommend a nonfoaming dispersible base), or unscented bath salts or crystals. The recommended dose for a full bath is ten to fifteen drops of essential oils. The maximum dose is thirty drops per bath; see table 14.

Table 14
Recommended Oils for Bath and Massage

Purpose	Essential oils	Suggested formula*		Effect
		Oil	No. of drops	
Relaxation/stress relief	Marjoram, orange, lavender, chamomile, tangerine, spikenard, neroli, ylang-ylang	Lavender Tangerine Marjoram Chamomile	3 3 3 1	Will induce a deep relaxation of the tissues, muscles, and joints and reestablish a good balance of energy
Energy/tissue firming	Lemon, peppermint, sage, thyme, rosemary, ginger, nutmeg, pepper	Peppermint Ginger Birch	4 3 3	General tonic for the endocrine glands and nervous system; tones the tissue (energetic massage)
Pain relief, sport massage, arthritis	Birch, rosemary, lavender, thyme, pine, chamomile, peppermint, camphor, juniper, ginger, nutmeg	Birch Rosemary Juniper Ginger	5 3 2 2	Will relieve rheumatic crisis, neuralgia, sores, and muscular aches
Circulation problems, cellulitis, water retention, obesity	Cypress, geranium lemon, thyme, grapefruit, juniper, angelica, fennel, birch	Grapefruit Lemon Juniper Cypress Red thyme	4 3 2 2 1	Will strengthen the circulatory system (lymphatic system, capillaries, veins) and fluidize, the blood; helpful for varicosis, hemorrhoids, obesity
Aphrodisiac	Jasmine, ylang-ylang, michelia flowers, cedarwood, geranium, vetiver, clary sage, pepper, cistus, sandalwood, patchouli	Ylang-ylang Jasmine Michelia flowers Sandalwood Patchouli	3 2 2 2 1	A delightful prelude or interlude
Nervousness	Mugwort, petitgrain, marjoram, neroli, rose, spikenard	Neroli Petitgrain Marjoram Spikenard	3 3 3 1	Mild nervous system sedative; encourages us to relax deeply and let go

*For one bath or to prepare 1 ounce (30 milliliters) of massage oil.

Aromatic Body Wrap

+ Lay a blanket on a comfortable horizontal surface (bed, carpet, massage table, etc.).
+ Cover the blanket with a plastic foil and place a large towel on top.
+ In a spray bottle, mix ten to fifteen drops of the appropriate blend of essential oils with 8 to 12 ounces (200 to 300 milliliters) of hot water and fifty to sixty drops of an emulsifier (any product that allows the dispersion of essential oils in water).
+ Shake well. Spray the oil mixture on the towel, shaking the bottle constantly.
+ Lie on the towel and wrap it around your whole body. Wrap the plastic foil and the blanket around you.
+ Breathe, relax, enjoy. . . . Enhance the experience with a quiet room, dim light, and nice, peaceful music.

Body wraps may also be done in "zones" or chakras. Soft cotton bandages are soaked in a bowl of hot water with ten to fifteen drops of essential oil blend, and the body is wrapped in sections. You can apply different oils on different parts of the body, one for each zone or body part. For instance, you could apply detoxifying oils on the lower body to activate toxin elimination and fight cellulitis and relaxing oils on the upper back and shoulders, where stress and tension tend to accumulate.

Dosage for Aromatic Body Wrap

Body wraps are a very safe way to apply essential oils. We strongly recommend the use of an

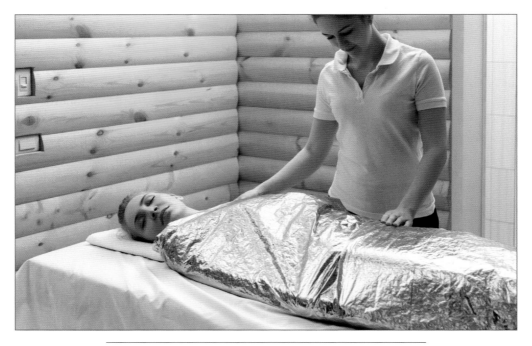

Aromatic body wrap

emulsifier to ensure proper dispersion of the essential oils. The recommended dose for a full body wrap is ten to fifteen drops. Maximum dose is fifty drops. The same cautions apply to body wraps as to massages (no ketones and only low doses of phenols). The most effective treatment is to follow the body wrap with a massage using the same blends.

Salt Glow

The salt glow (also called body gommage) is an exfoliating and detoxifying treatment that is very popular in Europe and Asia, especially Korea and Japan. For a body gommage treatment, mix 1 ounce of finely ground sea salt with ten to fifteen drops of essential oils (cypress, thyme, grapefruit, lemon, juniper, angelica, fennel). Moisten the salt with water or mix with a carrier oil or unscented lotion to obtain a paste that can be spread easily. Apply the preparation with your fingertips or with a washcloth or a loofa. Apply with circular movement on the entire body, especially the hips and thighs. A body gommage exfoliates dead cells from the outer skin layer, deep-cleanses the pores, activates capillary and lymphatic circulation, and stimulates the elimination of toxins. It is excellent for cellulitis or weight problems and can be done at home before the morning shower or before a bath. I recommend doing this two or three times a week.

Absorption, Distribution, and Bioavailability

Topical administration of essential oils, whether through massage, compress, bath, or body wrap, offers a relatively fast absorption time of fifteen

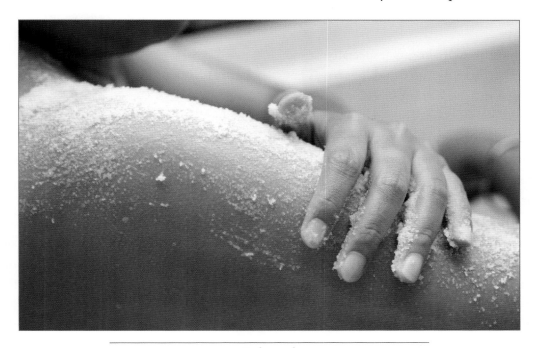

Salt scrub

to twenty minutes, with high availability of up to 90 percent. The quantities of essential oils actually administered can reach therapeutic levels.

Topically applied essential oils act primarily at the biophysical and energetic level. Topical use also produces olfactory stimulation and in this way can provoke emotional, mental, and spiritual action.

SKIN CARE USES OF ESSENTIAL OILS

Applied to the skin, essential oils regulate the activity of the capillaries and restore vitality to the tissues. According to Marguerite Maury (*The Secret of Life and Youth*), they are natural rejuvenating agents. They facilitate the elimination of waste matter and dead cells and promote the regeneration of new, healthy cells (cytophylactic power).

The most pleasant scents (especially flower oils) are the most useful for skin care. They can be used in facial steam baths, compresses, masks, and body wraps. They can be added to any kind of lotion, skin cream, gel, toilet water, or perfume. As a rule, never apply essential oils undiluted on the skin.

Floral waters are particularly well suited to skin care. Milder and easier to use than essential oils, they are recommended for sensitive and inflamed skins. Essential oils and floral waters have more or less the same indications. You can use plain floral water for compresses. You should use floral water instead of water in any skin care preparation. Finally, you will get

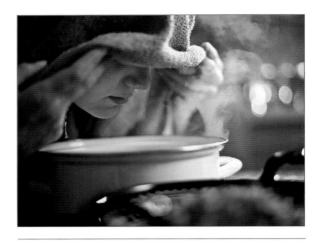

Facial sauna

an excellent facial tonic and astringent using floral water with a spray bottle (rose, sage, rosemary, lavender, cypress, etc.)—very refreshing. Floral waters retain the water-soluble plant chemicals, which do not appear in the finished essential oil. See table 15 (page 87) for a guide to oils for specific facial applications.

Facial Steam Bath

Add five to fifteen drops of essential oil to a bowl of hot water. Drape a large towel over your head and lower your face into the steam, letting it unclog your pores. Add a few drops every five minutes (ten to fifteen minutes total).

Facial Compresses

Add five drops of the appropriate blend of essential oils to a bowl of warm water (recommended dose, five drops; maximum dose, ten drops). Soak cotton or cloth in the blend. Apply to your face for five minutes. Resoak and reapply up to three times. Avoid phenolic oils.

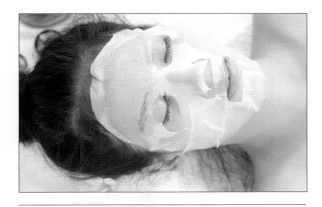

Facial compress

Eye Compresses

Use cotton pads soaked in warm floral water. For puffiness, irritation, and most eye compresses use chamomile floral water. For wrinkles around the eyes, use rose floral waters.

Masks

Facial masks are cleansing, nourishing, and revitalizing; they promote the elimination of waste material and stimulate local blood circulation. They can be soothing and moisturizing, depending on the ingredients. We strongly recommend using an emulsifier to ensure proper dispersion of the oils. Basic ingredients for a mask are clay, oatmeal, fruit or vegetable pulp, vegetable oil, floral water, and essential oils.

+ Put a few spoonfuls of clay and soaked oatmeal in a bowl; add the fruit (or vegetable) pulp and juice, a teaspoon of vegetable oil (wheat germ, for instance), and five drops of essential oils.
+ Stir, then add floral water, herb tea, or plain water until the mixture has the right consistency.
+ Apply to your face with your fingertips; let the mask dry for up to fifteen minutes, then gently remove it with a wet sponge.
+ Apply floral water to close the pores.
+ Normal skin needs a mask every one to two weeks.

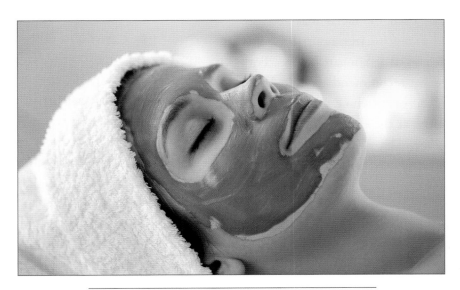

Facial mask

The recommended dose is five drops of essential oils in a mask, with fifteen drops being the maximum dose. In addition to oatmeal, clay, essential oils, and floral water, you can use:

For acne: cabbage, grape, yeast
For oily skin: cabbage, cucumber, lemon, grape, pear, strawberry
For dry skin: melon, carrot, avocado, wheat germ oil
For sensitive skin: honey, apple, grape, melon
For mature skin: apple, avocado, wheat germ oil
For normal skin: avocado, lemon, peach, wheat germ oil

Caution: Avoid phenolic oils, use only small amounts of green clay on dry skin, and use only small amounts of seaweed on sensitive skin.

Facial Oils

Facial oils can be used for facial massage, or they can be used as moisturizer, nourisher, and protectant at the end of a skin care session. For a facial massage we recommend using a base of sweet almond oil or hazelnut oil. For facial nourishment, to use at the end of the skin care session, we recommend hazelnut oil (90 percent) with vitamin E oil (2 percent), evening primrose oil (4 percent), and borage oil (4 percent) blended together.

For a facial oil we recommend the following blend as a base (for a 1-ounce or 30-milliliter preparation).

Hazelnut oil: 8 ml
Squalene: 8 ml
Jojoba: 8 ml
Helio-carrot: 3 ml
Evening primrose, borage, or rosa mosceta (or a combination of the three): 2 ml
Vitamin E: 1 ml

Dosage

The recommended concentration for facial oils is 3 to 4 percent, or thirty to forty drops of essential oil in 1 ounce (30 milliliters) of carrier oil. The maximum concentration is 8 percent, or eighty drops in 1 ounce (30 milliliters) of carrier oil.

Caution for Use of Essential Oils in Skin Care

General Cautions

+ As a general rule, never apply pure essential oils directly to the face.
+ Never use essential oils around the eyes.
+ Avoid using phenolic oils (clove, oregano, savory, red thyme) on the face.
+ In sunny climates do not use bergamot oil, and use only low concentrations of citrus oils (lemon, lime, orange, tangerine). All citrus oils, especially bergamot, increase photosensitivity and may cause sunspots.
+ On dry skin do not use phenolic or drying oils, such as eucalyptus or the oils rich in terpenes (pine and fir).
+ On inflamed and sensitive skin lower the essential oil concentration, and do not use phenolic oils.

Table 15
Essential Oils for Skin Care

Skin type/problem	Essential oils
Normal skin	Clary sage, geranium, lavender, ylang-ylang, rosewood
Dry skin	Spanish sage, clary sage, cedarwood, sandalwood, rose, palmarosa, carrot seed
Oily skin	Lavender, lemon, geranium, basil, camphor, frankincense, rosemary, ylang-ylang
Inflamed skin	German chamomile, helichrysum, clary sage, lavender, myrrh, patchouli, carrot seed, floral waters
Sensitive skin	Roman chamomile, neroli, rosewood, floral waters
Acne	Cajeput, tea tree, eucalyptus, juniper, lavender, palmarosa, niaouli
Eczema	Cedarwood, German chamomile, lavender, sage, patchouli, rose, benzoin
Rejuvenation	Benzoin, frankincense, sandalwood, cedarwood, geranium, lavender, myrrh, rosemary, carrot seed
Seborrhea	Bergamot, lavender, Spanish sage, cypress, patchouli
Broken capillaries	Rose, ylang-ylang
Wrinkles	Fennel, lemon, palmarosa, myrrh, frankincense, patchouli, clary sage, carrot seed

Lotions, Potions, Body Oils, Bath Oils, Ointments

Numerous stories of scented ointments or potions, from the remotest antiquity to the Renaissance, from the Holy Bible to the most lascivious mythological tales, are recounted. For example, Mary Magdalene gave a foot rub to Christ with precious ointments, and according to venomous tongues, Cleopatra owed her seductive power to her secret potions rather than to her beauty. Lotions, potions, creams, and ointments would contain the following basic ingredients.

A solidifier (lanolin or beeswax)
An oil (sweet almond, avocado, hazelnut, jojoba, or whatever is best for your skin type; see the section on carrier oils in chapter 10)
Distillates or flower water (or distilled water)
A blend of essential oils

The kind of product you create will depend on the proportion of the ingredients (for a cream, for example, you might use 1 ounce beeswax, 4 ounces vegetable oil, 2 ounces water, and ¼ ounce essential oils). Melt the solidifier in a double boiler, and slowly add the oil and water, stirring continuously. Let the mixture cool a bit until it starts to thicken, then add the essential oils and stir thoroughly. Store in tightly closed opaque jars.

Hair Care

Mix ¼ ounce of essential oil in 16 ounces of a good shampoo or hair conditioner.

Dry hair: Cade, cedarwood
Hair loss: Cedarwood, juniper, lavender, rosemary, sage
Normal hair: Chamomile, lavender, ylang-ylang
Oily hair: Lemongrass, rosemary
Scalp diseases: Cedarwood, rosemary, sage, cade
Dandruff: Rosemary, cedarwood, cade

For a scalp rub use flower water or ¼ ounce of essential oils mixed in 4 ounces of grain alcohol or sweet almond oil.

SAFETY GUIDELINES

Essential oils are very powerful substances that should be treated with respect; they are highly concentrated plant extracts and should not be abused. Each drop is equivalent to at least 1 ounce of plant material. Therefore it is always important to carefully respect the doses (see table 16). In most cases, essential oils are more potent in infinitesimal doses. Increasing the dosage will not usually increase efficacy.

Some oils, such as the phenolic oils, can be irritating, while others, like the ketones, can be toxic. Proper dosage is critical. The recommended dosage for each type of application and the maximum dosage for safe use are listed in table 16.

Table 16
Recommended Dosages for the Use of Essential Oils in Skin Care

Application	%	Drops in 1 oz	2 oz	4 oz	Milliliters in 100 ml	Use
Massage						
Full-body massage	1.50	15	30	60	1.50	15 ml (1½ oz) for full body
Local massage	3.00	30	60	120	3.00	10 to 15 drops on area
Topical application	6.00	60	120	240	6.00	5 drops on point
Bath						
Foaming bath gel	3.00	30	60	120	3.00	15 ml (½ oz) in one bath
Bath oil	5.00	50	100	200	5.00	10 ml (1⅓ oz) in one bath
Bath salts and crystals	3.00	30	60	120	3.00	15 ml (1½ oz) in one bath
Skin						
Facial steam						5 to 10 drops in hot water
Compress						5 to 10 drops in warm water
Mask	2.00	20	40	80	2.00	10 g (⅓ oz) per mask
Facial oil	2.00	20	40	80	2.00	3 to 5 drops for facial massage

CONCLUSION

When you first step into the essential oil world, you might be a little bit surprised, or even slightly turned off. Your olfactory system will have to be reeducated, or rather detoxified. After years of neglect and abuse with junk perfumes, your nose might not be able to fully appreciate the richness of natural fragrances. Just like when you change your eating habits from junk food to a more healthy diet, you cannot really appreciate the full flavor of a lettuce leaf, a plain radish, or a bowl of brown rice. But when you start to detoxify, your taste greatly improves and refines, and soon you do not want to come back to junk again.

Then the power of fragrances moves you every day; you play with them, dance with them, create with them. They connect you to the quintessence of the realm of plants. As William Langham writes in *The Garden of Health* (1579), they will "make thee glad, merry, gracious and well-beloved of all men."

EIGHT

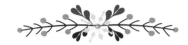

Essential Oil Classifications

Plants are classified in botanical families according to the structure of their flowers. But this classification goes beyond the flower itself. Each plant of the same family appears like a variation of the basic model of the type: same leaf and seed structure, similar rhythm (in space and time), and similar chemical composition.

With Goethe, the anthroposophists believe in an archetypal plant that exhibits the structural potentialities of the vegetable kingdom and manifests itself through different degrees of differentiation in families, species, and chemotypes. In this system each type expressed by the botanical families represents a certain degree of evolution of the archetypal model—a certain level of actualization of its potentialities, from the primitive of the Equisetaceae (horsetail) to the most evolved of the Rosaceae (rose, apple, etc.). Differentiation of the type generates the species (or genus), which is then further differentiated in subspecies and chemotypes. In the anthroposophic vision, inspired by the works

of Paracelsus and the study of homeopathy, the physical aspect of the plants and the nature of their interactions with the environment are correlated with their medicinal properties. A type of therapeutic activity is attributed to each botanical family, variations being related to each plant of the family. This approach is quite rich and accurate. It is fairly consistent with the more classical systems of herbal therapy and aromatherapy: there are some obvious similarities between the recommended uses of plants in the same family.

While a wildcrafter in southern France, I experienced the accuracy of such a vision. In some powerful experiences of intimate communication with plants, I felt that the plants introduced themselves to me and I could tell the medicinal properties or even the names of plants that I had never seen before. More generally, I found that careful observation of the plant and its environment told me much about its activity.

At any rate, classification of essential oils by botanical families tells more about their therapeutic activity than a mere alphabetical classification, and that will be my approach to this chapter. I hope that this gives my readers a better understanding of aromatherapy.

SYNTHETICS VERSUS NATURAL: DOES IT MAKE SCENTS?

Many people think that molecules produced through the processes of life are more active in a living context (such as medicine) than their synthetic counterparts are, although they cannot really be chemically differentiated from their natural cousins. There is even growing evidence that this belief is well founded. Along the same line of thought, a natural extract is often found to be more efficient than its main active ingredient.

Is it possible that molecules have some kind of memory? That they store the information pertaining to their history? That life shares a common pool of memories? That natural molecules are more accurate in dealing with living organisms because they have stored living memory? If so, a natural molecule could "know" how to deal with other living molecules. Each molecule belonging to a given extract would have a memory of its companions and could predictably be more efficient when not separated from these companions.

THE CONCEPT OF MORPHOGENETIC FIELDS

When bicycles were first invented, it took people months to learn how to ride them. How long did it take your kids to learn how to ride their bikes? A few hours? Two days? When the first cars were invented, most people were too scared to even think about driving them. Now the average teenager learns how to drive in very little time. When Einstein introduced the theory of relativity, years passed before a handful of people could figure it out. Currently relativity is taught in college. How long did it take you to learn how to use a computer? How long did it take your kids? When you look at up-to-date college textbooks, how often do you feel that you haven't any clue to what they are all about?

According to Rupert Sheldrake, all these phenomena can be accounted for by the concept of morphogenetic fields, a theory that we can manifest what we create in our thoughts just by envisioning. To put it simply, a morphogenetic field can be viewed as a landscape, with mountains, valleys, plains, riverbeds, and so on. Each valley and each riverbed corresponds to flows of information, all interconnected. A totally new input of information can be viewed as a small furrow being traced somewhere in the landscape. The more this information is used, the deeper its furrow becomes, and the more likely it will be to attract new information, until it resembles a valley or a main stream. Learning a new technique, for instance, deepens the corresponding furrow. The greater the number of people who learn this technique, the deeper the furrow, and the easier it becomes for other people to learn the technique.

Of course a new furrow is generated only when the landscape is ready for it. This would account for the fact that very often, whenever the ground is ready for a new discovery, several people will make this discovery at the same time.* Conversely, whenever an area of the morphogenetic field does not flow, it becomes locally stagnant, and sediment accumulates. Thus valleys are filled up, riverbeds disappear, and information is buried because of disuse.

The concept of the morphogenetic field is an excellent tool for describing all the processes of evolution, whether evolution of the universe, evolution of species, cultural evolution, or personal evolution. It helps us understand how patterns are created. For example, positive thinking is a personal application of the morphogenetic field; it can act as the path to achieving one's goals by attracting positive experience. The more we imagine ourselves achieving success, the more successful we become. This is why I am an incurable optimist and why I think that pessimists are always wrong, especially when they are right.

Botanical families can be viewed as deep valleys in the vegetal morphogenetic field, dividing into the rivers of species and the streams of subspecies of chemotypes. Each of these valleys, rivers, and streams has been generated throughout the ages in close interaction with the local and global environment (other fami-

lies and species and the ecosystems supporting them, including microorganisms, animals, and humans).

We can see how the concept of the morphogenetic field is in total agreement with the Gaia hypothesis. Our planet is a living organism. Humanity has brought consciousness to this organism—for a purpose, undoubtedly. This purpose cannot be the destruction of the planet. As conscious cells of this organism, we have a responsibility to take care of our planet. Otherwise, we behave like a virus in a sick body, and the organism will try to get rid of us. A lose-lose situation.

Our planet, the body we all live in together, is presently going through an acute toxic crisis. For those of you familiar with natural healing, this means that our planet will most probably need to go through a dramatic discharge process. But this is an emergency. No economic or other consideration can prevail against this absolute necessity. There is now an enormous worldwide awareness of this crisis. This can be viewed as a natural defense mechanism of our planet. We must capitalize on this movement and start acting now. We can do it, individually and collectively.

BACK TO THE BOTANICAL FAMILIES

Botanical Families and the Gaia Hypothesis

The vegetable kingdom appeared on our planet long before the animal kingdom. Through evolution, from the primitive moss or fern, it gradually

---

*Interestingly enough, in the late 1970s my research into logic and the theory of information came very close to the ideas that Rupert Sheldrake was developing (I talked about field of forms; he talks about morphogenetic fields). I presented a paper at the University of California at Berkeley in 1980 to explain my theories. I was not aware of Sheldrake at that time, nor was he aware of my work.

differentiated to generate the thousands of species that we now know. This evolution was at first independent of the animal kingdom (but maybe it was preparing the ground for it—by producing oxygen, for instance). Then, when the first animals appeared on our planet (and they appeared because the morphogenetic field was ready for them), the two realms evolved in close interaction. For example, more and more vegetable species came to depend on insects for pollination. And, of course, animals were totally dependent on plants for their subsistence.

It is not unreasonable to think that this interaction went very far; plants were not only food for the animal kingdom but were also medicine. Animals provided fertilizers; they carried the seeds and buried them, moved the ground with their feet, and trimmed the bushes. If the Gaia hypothesis is well founded—and I believe that it is—and if our planet can be viewed as a living organism, this is not surprising.

Certain plants became specialized in their interaction with the animal kingdom. Human intervention further accentuated this process; the plants that are now cultivated domestically have been "created" through a long selection process. The varieties of corn, wheat, apples, or potatoes that we buy in our supermarkets do not exist in the wild—they were produced through genetic breeding.

The study of botanical families, by going from the global (the vegetable kingdom) to the particular (the species and the subspecies) through the differentiation process (the botanical families), gives us a better understanding

of and appreciation for our living planet. Each plant has accumulated through the millions of years of its history the living memory of the vegetable kingdom, the memory of its family, the memory of its genus and its species. All this information is here for us to share and respect. This is an ongoing miracle.

The Plant's Domain of Creativity

When we look at a planet from the perspective of the botanical family, we can learn a lot from the family itself. We also can learn from the part of the plant where its creativity is the most developed, and, in studying aromatherapy, where its essential oil is produced.

Each family seems to have a privileged domain of creativity. The Lamiaceae and Myrtacea produce their essential oils mostly in the leaves. The rose produces them in the flower; the citruses in the flower, the fruit, and the leaves; the Burseraceae in their exudate; and so on.

Evolution Involution

Each plant goes from the physical sphere, with the germ and then the roots, through the vital sphere with the leaves, and to the astral sphere with the flower in a natural evolution process. It then creates its fruit or seed in an involution back to the physical world.

Essential oils produced in the roots (angelica, vetiver) tend to have a very grounding energy; they have a foodlike quality to them. They are not very refined, but they usually are potent stimulants of the vital functions (especially digestion) of the organism. Typically, they are recommended for anemia.

The plant's leaf system corresponds to its vital body. Essential oils produced in the leaves (eucalyptus, niaouli, peppermint, etc.) have a strong affinity with the prajna energy and the respiratory system. They tone the vital body. Excessive development of the leaf system of a plant is a sign of etheric imbalance that can produce toxicity (as in some Umbelliferae).

The flower is the plant's ultimate achievement. Only the most spiritually evolved plants (such as the rose) can fully create at this level. The production of fragrance is then a sign of intense astral activity. Although the essential oils are found in extremely small amounts in the flowers, their fragrances are typically very intense, although refined in nature. The plants with the most intense floral creativity rarely produce any significant fruit or seed. These plants' creativity is exhausted with the fragrance, and their creation does not belong to the physical plant any longer. Such fragrances have a tendency to be exhilarating (jasmine) or even intoxicating (narcissus).

The essential oils of flowers are then usually very refined and subtle but very hard to extract. They often are too far removed from the physical sphere to be extracted through steam distillation. (Neroli and rose are an exception, as

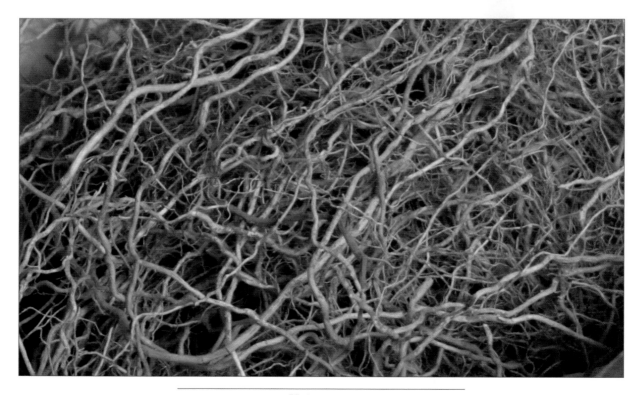

Vetiver roots

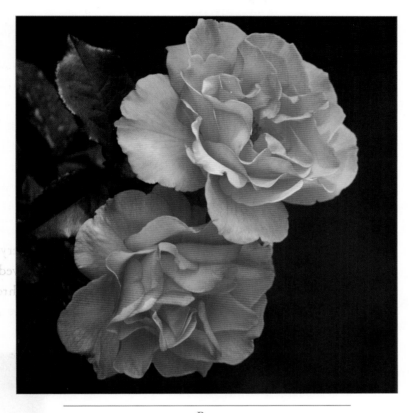

Rose

they are particularly well-balanced plants; they both produce edible fruits: oranges and rose hips, respectively.) Very sensitive to temperature, their molecules break apart when exposed to heat. Some of them can be extracted by solvents (jasmine, tuberose, narcissus).

The oils produced in the seed bring us back fully into the physical world, being less sophisticated, more humble, and straightforward (citrus fruits, anise, fennel, coriander). They are invigorating and fortifying and show a strong affinity with the digestive system (especially those seeds that are food or spices).

Trees and bushes also have the ability to create oils in their wood (sandalwood, cedarwood). Such oils are centering and equilibrating. Here the creative process is drawn into the heart of the wood. These oils have the power to open our consciousness to higher spheres without making us lose control. They are particularly suited to rituals, meditation, and yoga.

Finally, many trees and bushes (myrrh, frankincense, conifers, cistus) produce odorous resins or gums. These essential oils have a strong affinity for the glandular system; they control secretions and demonstrate cosmetic and healing properties (skin care, wounds, ulcers).

NINE

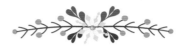

The Essential Oils in Botanical Families

ANONACEAE

Exuberant Fruity Creativity of Tropical Living Fossils

Commonly known as the custard apple family or soursop family, Annonaceae is the largest family of the magnolia order (Magnoliales). It is one of the most primitive families of angiosperms (flowering plants) and can be considered a living fossil.

Found mainly in the tropics all around the globe, especially in rain forests, the family consists of trees, shrubs, and, more rarely, lianas. Although the bark, leaves, flowers, and roots of many species are aromatic and used as spices and in folk medicine, only ylang-ylang essential oil is produced commercially.

Many species produce large, pulpy fruits, such as guanabana (soursop), cherimoya, atemoya (custard apple), rollinia, sugar apple (sweetsop), pawpaw, kepel apple, pond apple, marolo, and bush banana.

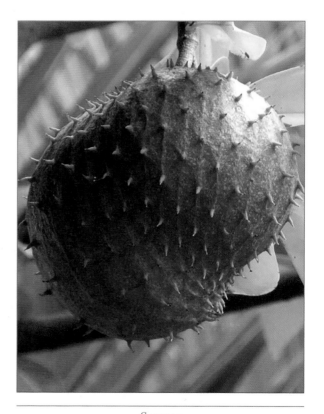

Soursop

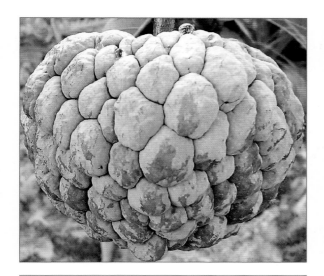

Sweetsop

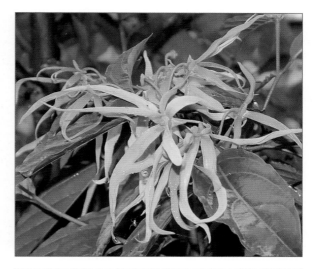

Ylang-ylang

The family exudes an exuberant creativity that allowed it to survive many mass extinctions and manifests in the production of its often gigantic and delicious fruits and the aromatic and medicinal substances in its bark, leaves, and flowers.

Ylang-Ylang (*Unona odoratissima*)

🍂 Primarily produced in Réunion, the Comoro Islands, Madagascar, Java, Sumatra, and the Philippines

🍂 Fragrance: Sweet, voluptuous, and exotic (even sickening for some people)

Ylang-ylang is closely related to cananga (*Cananga odorata*). The two could in fact be the same tree; the slight difference between the essences would then depend on the country of production and the method of distillation.

The distillation of the flowers is a delicate operation that lasts for days; it yields up to six different qualities, from extra-superior to fifth grade. The "complete" (i.e., the whole oil) should be used for aromatherapy. The oil is yellowish and syrupy and makes a good fragrance fixative.

Ylang-ylang, whose name means "flower of flowers," is a tree growing up to 60 feet high that produces beautiful yellow flowers. In Indonesia people spread them on the bed of newly married couples on their wedding night. In the Molucca Islands people soak ylang-ylang and cucuma flowers in coconut to prepare an ointment called *borri-borri,* which they use for skin care, hair care, and skin disease and to prevent fever. According to R. W. Moncrieff, "Ylang-ylang oil soothes and inhibits anger born of frustration."

Supremely exotic, ylang-ylang has the soothing, sedative, slightly euphoric, even lascivious quality of extreme fire and water, the luxurious laziness of tropical islands. It is used especially as a perfume, in baths, for massage, and in cosmetics. It also has a soothing effect on the skin and is recommended for oily skin. Ylang-ylang's use as the distinctive scent of legendary perfume Chanel N°5 propelled it to fame in 1921, and it has since been used in numerous perfumes.

Medicinal properties: Hypotensive; aphrodisiac; antidepressant, sedative, euphoric; antiseptic (for intestinal infections)
Indications: Tachycardia, palpitations; hypertension, hyperpnea; depression, nervous tension, insomnia; impotence, frigidity; skin care

APIACEAE (UMBELLIFERAE)
Plants of the Air Element

Essential oils of this family include angelica, aniseed, caraway, carrot, coriander, cumin, fennel, and lovage. Other oils of interest are *Ammi visnaga,* dill, asafetida, celery, galbanum, and parsley.

This family is characterized by the extreme

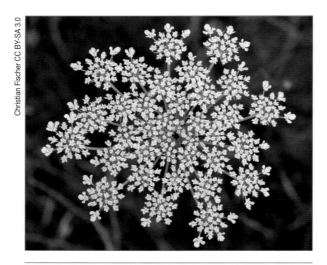

Christian Fischer CC BY-SA 3.0

Wild carrot

division of the leaves, ending up in an aerial explosion in such plants as fennel and anise. The leaf is the origin of interaction and confrontation between air and water, light and darkness.

Apiaceae obviously are very sensitive to this confrontation. The interaction of air, light, water, and earth through these extremely ramified leaves gives birth, in a contraction process, to a strong root or vigorous rhizome, which stays underground for a year or more. This subterranean organ draws the cosmic forces into the ground. Then vegetation grows rapidly in a radiating explosion until it reaches the final bouquet of the inflorescence, with its radiating umbel—each branch of the umbel splitting again in umbellules.

The special interaction of this family with the air element is further emphasized by the plants' ability to incorporate air within themselves in hollow stems, hollow seeds, and even hollow rhizomes.

In the archetypal plant the interaction between the plant's etheric organism and the surrounding astral forces takes place in the flower area. This process is manifested in the colors and fragrance of the flower and the formation of nectar. Apiaceae attract cosmic forces in the leaves, the stem, and even the rhizome. Their aromatic substances are therefore heavier, harsher, and less refined than floral scents.

Apiaceae, in fact, start their fructification process in the leaves, or even the root. They produce some of the most tasty vegetables (carrot, celery, fennel) and condiments (parsley, coriander, chervil, anise, cumin, caraway, etc.).

In addition to this descending movement, there is also an ascending movement of mucilages and gums, another characteristic of the family. The therapeutic action of Apiaceae is then easy to understand. First, they have an affinity for the digestive system (especially the intestine); also, they have a strong effect on the secretions and the glandular system. Finally, they are useful in respiratory diseases.

According to Robert Tisserand's *Aromatherapy to Heal and Tend the Body*, "Tissue regeneration in the livers of rats has been demonstrated in the essential oils, in particular the four seed oils—cumin, fennel, celery and parsley" (which all belong to the Apiaceae family). Carrot seed oil has been used successfully to fight against the aging skin process.

Type of action: Accumulation/excretion, elimination; secretion (diuretic, sudorific, expectorant); regulation of the aerial processes in the organism (carminative, antispasmodic); tissue regeneration
Domain of action: Digestive system (especially intestines), glandular system, respiratory system
Indications: Digestive and intestinal problems, accumulation of gas; spasms (digestive, respiratory, circulatory); glandular problems

Angelica (*Angelica archangelica*)

- Primarily produced in Belgium, France, and Poland
- Essential oil is obtained from seeds or roots; it is almost colorless
- Fragrance: Balsamic, nicely aromatic, and slightly musky

Several varieties of angelica grow in northern Europe, mainly *Angelica sylvestris* (wild) and *Angelica archangelica* (domestic, cultured). The plant was highly valued by physicians of the Renaissance. Paracelsus reported that it was of great help during the epidemic of pestilence in Milan in 1510.

This vigorous, prolific plant of the air element (with a hollow stem) grows in deep humid soils and rather cool climates. (It grows wild by streams and irrigation canals.) Therefore it is a typical plant of elimination. It helps eliminate toxins, purify the blood and lymph, and stimulate the glandular system. It is recommended in cases of weakness and nervousness, for convalescents, and for old people.

Medicinal properties: Depurative, sudorific; stomachic, digestive, aperitive; stimulant, tonic, cephalic, revitalizing
Indications: Nervous afflictions related to the digestive system (cramps, spasms, aerophagia, digestive migraine); weakness of stomach; asthenia, anemia, anorexia, rickets, neurovegetative cardiopathies; lung diseases (bronchitis, flu, pneumonia, pleuresy); gout (use in compresses and gentle massage)

Aniseed (*Pimpinella anisum*)

- Primarily produced in Spain, Egypt, North Africa, and countries of the former Soviet Union
- Essential oil is distilled from the seeds; it is slightly yellow

Mentioned in the Vedas and the Bible, anise was considered one of the main medicinal plants in China, India, Egypt, Greece, and Rome. According to Pythagorus, it is an excellent carminative and appetite stimulant.

Unlike most Apiaceae, anise grows flowers and seeds in its first year. Only in a very dry climate can the seeds fully ripen. The forces of warmth are thus condensed in these small aniseeds, the taste of which is aqueous and fiery. The medicinal properties of anise are then the same as those of most plants of the type, but its antispasmodic expectorant power is accentuated, with a narcotic or even stupefying effect.

Medicinal properties: Stomachic, carminative, antispasmodic; general stimulant (digestive, respiratory, cardiac); galactogogue; diuretic; aphrodisiac; stupefying at high doses
Indications: Nervous dyspepsia, aerophagia, gas accumulation, digestive migraines; insufficient milk (nursing mothers); impotence, frigidity; epilepsy

Caraway (*Carum carvi*)

🌿 Primarily produced in northern Europe
🌿 Essential oil is distilled from the seeds; it is yellowish

Caraway seed is used in pastries and delicatessen foods in northern Europe and the Arabic countries. Its medicinal properties are very similar to those of aniseed.

Medicinal properties: Carminative; antispasmodic; general stimulant (digestive, respiratory, cardiac); diuretic

Indications: Digestive and intestinal troubles; aerophagia, gas accumulation, fermentations, nervous dyspepsia, digestive migraine; scabies, mange (dogs)

Carrot (*Daucus carota*)

🌿 Primarily produced in France, Egypt, and India
🌿 Essential oil is distilled from the seeds; it is slightly yellow
🌿 Fragrance: Characteristic (carrotlike)

Carrot has been used since the sixteenth century as a carminative, diuretic, and hepatic and for skin diseases.

Medicinal properties: Depurative, hepatic; emmenagogue; diuretic
Indications: Jaundice, hepatobiliary disorders; skin diseases; facilitates menstruation and conception

Coriander (*Coriandrum sativum*)

🌿 Primarily produced in North Africa, Spain, and countries of the former Soviet Union
🌿 Essential oil is distilled from the seeds; it is slightly yellow
🌿 Fragrance: Anise-y, musky, and aromatic

Seeds of coriander found in Egyptian sepulchers prove that it was already in use by the time of Ramses II. Theophrasta, Hippocrates, Galen, and Pliny talk about its properties as a stimulant, carminative, and digestive.

Medicinal properties and indications: Same as all Apiaceae (aerophagia, digestion, flatulence, spasms); stupefying at high doses

Cumin (*Cuminum cyminum*)

- Primarily produced in North Africa and the Far East
- Essential oil is distilled from the seeds; it is slightly yellow
- Fragrance: Bitter, anise-y, and aromatic

Native to Egypt, cumin is a close relative of coriander. It was a traditional spice in the Middle East and is one of the ingredients of curry. It is an excellent digestive stimulant, though it should be used with great care as it can provoke skin irritation.

Medicinal properties and indications: Same as all Apiaceae (aerophagia, digestion, flatulence, spasms)

Fennel (*Foeniculum vulgare*)

- Primarily produced in Spain, North Africa, India, and Japan
- Essential oil is distilled from the seeds; it is yellowish
- Fragrance: Strong, anise-y, and camphoric

Fennel is used in the cuisine and medicine of India, Egypt, and China. In the Middle Ages people used it to prevent witchcraft and as a protection against evil spirits.

Medicinal properties: Aperitive, stomachic, carminative; emmenagogue, galactogogue; diuretic; antispasmodic; laxative
Indications: Dyspepsia, flatulence, digestive problems, aerophagia; amenorrhea, menopausal problems; insufficient milk; oliguria, obesity, kidney stones

Lovage (*Levisticum officinale*)

- Primarily produced in France and Belgium
- Essential oil is distilled from the roots; it is slightly yellow
- Fragrance: Musky and earthy

Medicinal properties: Intestinal and kidney stimulant; diuretic; drainer, detoxifier
Indications: Kidney afflictions (cystitis, nephritis, albuminuria, etc.); water retention, edema; intestinal fermentation

ASTERACEAE (COMPOSITAE)
Realization, Organization, and Structure

Essential oils of this family include chamomile, everlasting, mugwort, and tarragon. Other oils of interest are arnica, calendula, tansy, yarrow, and wormwood.

The Asteraceae are characterized by their inflorescence, a collection of small flowers forming a unique superior entity. This basic simple structure is able to generate such a diversity that, with about eight hundred genera and thirteen thousand species, the Asteraceae constitute the largest botanical family.

Unlike orchids, another large family with amazing floral variations, Asteraceae grow all over the world in large settlements. They live in almost every terrestrial zone, except the far north and the tropical forest, from seashores to mountaintops, from desert to swamps, with a preference for open spaces widely exposed to light, such as meadows and steppes.

Very adaptive and intensely associated with

light, Asteraceae live primarily in the floral sphere. Because they embody a perfect balance of etheric and astral forces, the therapeutic activity of the plants of this family shows great diversity.

Chamomile (*Anthemis nobilis, A. mixta, Chamomilla matricaria, Ormenis multicaulis*)

- Primarily produced in France, Morocco, Spain, and Egypt
- Essential oil is distilled from the flowers; the oil of *Anthemis nobilis* (Roman chamomile) and *Anthemis mixta* is yellow, while the oils of *Chamomilla matricaria* (German chamomile) is light blue and *Ormenis multicaulis* (blue chamomile) is dark blue, owing to the presence of azulene

- Fragrance: Refreshing and aromatic
- Used in perfumery, cosmetics, and pharmacy

Dedicated to the sun by the Egyptians for its febrifuge properties, chamomile is probably one of the oldest known medicinal plants. It was traditionally regarded as the plants' physician— that is, it was thought to keep other plants in good health.

Interest in chamomile has recently been revived with the discovery of azulene, an excellent anti-inflammatory agent, which is not present in the fresh flower but is formed when the plant is distilled. Many different botanical species around the world are called chamomile. Roman chamomile (*Anthemis nobilis*) and German chamomile (*Chamomilla matricaria*) are the most commonly used in herbology. The oil called chamomile mixta or "wild

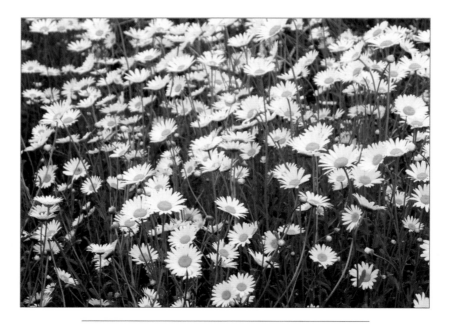

Chamomile

chamomile" (*Anthemis mixta*) is distilled from the wild in southern Spain and Morocco. Blue chamomile is distilled in Morocco and Egypt. A pineapple-scented chamomile grows throughout the United States (but its essential oil has not been distilled, as far as I know). Other varieties of chamomile grow in different parts of the world but are used only locally.

Roman chamomile is an excellent calming and soothing essential oil and a liver stimulant. German chamomile (whose species name, *matricaria,* is German for "mother herb") is especially indicated for female disorders (painful or irregular period, excessive loss of blood, hemorrhage). The whole plant is radiantly aerial; each beam terminates in a white-and-gold flower with a bulging receptacle, which encloses a drop of air. This flower manifests a subdued ardor, an appeased and soothing flame. (See also appendix 1 for the differences between the chamomiles.)

Chamomile likes light; it grows on roadsides and in open fields in light sandy soils. Its affinity for the air element and its particular connection with the aerial sphere indicate its strong therapeutic action on the abnormal astral processes in the human organism. It is beneficent against spasms, convulsions, hypersensitivity, menstruation troubles, colic, and neuralgic aches.

Medicinal properties: Anti-inflammatory (especially German chamomile); antispasmodic, mild nervous sedative (helpful for children), anticonvulsive, antidepressant; emmenagogue; antianemic; febrifuge, sudorific; hepatic, cholagogue; antiseptic; analgesic; stimulant of leukocytosis; cicatrizant, vulnerary; local vasoconstrictor

Indications: Infectious diseases, fever; anemia; inflammation; migraine, depression, headache, convulsions, insomnia, vertigo, irritability, hysteria; dysmenorrhea, amenorrhea, vaginitis, menopausal problems, vulvar pruritus; liver and spleen congestion; painful digestion, digestive problems of children, gastralgia, gastritis; ulcers (stomach, intestines); colic, colitis; neuralgia, rheumatism; teething pains, toothache, gingivitis; earache; wounds, burns, boils, urticaria, dermatitis, skin diseases, skin care; conjunctivitis; pronounced effect on the mind and nervous system (anger, oversensitivity, temper tantrums in children)

Everlasting (*Helichrysum italicum*)

- Primarily produced in southern France, Italy, and Yugoslavia
- Essential oil is distilled from the whole plant; it is yellowish
- Fragrance: Strongly aromatic

Everlasting is a fairly new oil in aromatherapy. My friend Gilles Garcin, with whom I used to distill wild lavender in the southern Alps of France, might very well have been the first to have distilled the plant for aromatherapy (incidentally, he used Henri Viaud's distillery). It has proved to be valuable for wounds and bruises.

Medicinal properties: Anti-inflammatory, antiphlogistic (according to Kurt Schnaubelt, it is even more potent than blue chamomile); cell regenerator

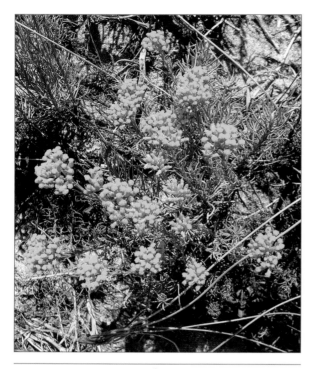

Everlasting

Indications: Hemorrhage; bruises, trauma; open wounds

Mugwort (*Artemisia vulgaris, A. herba-alba*)

- Primarily produced in Morocco and North Africa
- The oil is distilled from the whole plant; it is yellowish brown
- Fragrance: Strongly aromatic, and slightly musky

Named after the goddess Artemis (or Diana), protectress of virgins, mugwort had an ancient reputation as a specific for female cycles. It was also a magical plant, known to increase psychic power.

Related organs: Female reproductive system

Medicinal properties: Emmenagogue (abortive at high doses), regulator of the feminine cycle; antispasmodic; cholagogue, tonic, aperitive; vermifuge

Indications: Menstrual troubles (amenorrhea, dysmenorrhea; scanty, insufficient, or excessive periods); hysteria, convulsion, epilepsy, nervous vomiting; ascariasis, oxyuriasis

Tarragon (*Artemisia dracunculus*)

- Primarily produced in France, the United States, and Belgium
- Essential oil is distilled from the whole plant; it is almost colorless
- Fragrance: Anise-y and aromatic

Medicinal properties: Stimulant of the digestive system (stomach and intestine); antispasmodic; carminative, aperitive; vermifuge

Indications: Dyspepsia, hiccups; dystonia, weak digestion; aerophagia, fermentation; intestinal parasites

BETULACEAE
The Pain-Relief Family

Betulaceae are deciduous nut-bearing trees and shrubs distributed in temperate and subarctic areas of the Northern Hemisphere as well as in tropical mountains. The family can be divided into two subfamilies: Betuloideae, with the genera *Betula* (birch) and *Alnus* (alder), and Coryloideae, which includes *Corylus avellana*, the common hazelnut.

Birch and alder produce hard, pale red-

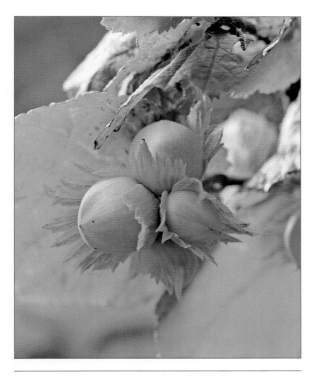

Common hazelnut

brown wood sold for furniture, woodenware, veneer, and flooring. Birch leaves, bark, and sap have been traditionally used in folk and herbal medicine for arthritis, rheumatism, urinary tract conditions, skin rashes, and hair loss.

Birch (*Betula lenta, B. alleghaniensis, and B. nigra*)

- Primarily produced in the northeastern United States
- Essential oil is distilled from the bark; it is clear to yellowish
- Fragrance: Balsamic, sweet, and warm
- Used in liniments and unguents for muscular and articular aches

Birch essential oil can be up to 98 percent methyl salicylate and therefore is quite often adulterated with the latter product. Two varieties of birch essential oil have been differentiated: northern birch essential oils, produced in Pennsylvania, Vermont, and New Hampshire (which apparently is no longer produced), and southern birch essential oil, produced in the southern part of the Appalachian mountains.

Wintergreen oil is similar to birch oil in its composition; essential oil sold as wintergreen is often methyl salicylate or birch essential oil.

Related organs: Kidneys, joints
Medicinal properties: Diuretic; analgesic; purifying, draining (lymphatic), cleansing

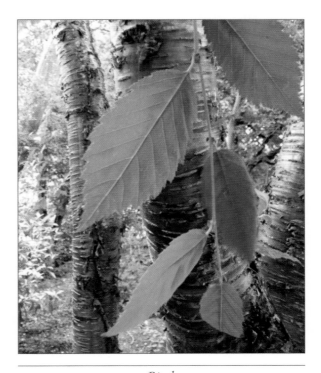

Birch

Indications: Rheumatism, arthritis, muscular and articular pains (one of the best remedies); kidney and urinary tract disorders (cystitis, stones, mucous discharge, dropsy); autointoxication caused by poor elimination of urea, cholesterol, glucose; skin diseases

BURSERACEAE
The Sacred Family

The essential oils of this family include elemi, frankincense, and myrrh. Another oil of interest in the family is copal.

Burseraceae grow in desert tropical areas where the intense cosmic activity promotes the formation of gum and etheric oils. The small boswellia tree (the source of frankincense), the most characteristic representative of the type, grows in the Arabian peninsula, in the most extreme climate of the planet. It is surrounded by a thin cloud of essential oil, which filters the sun's rays and freshens the air around it—hence its strong anti-inflammatory action. Burseraceae act against inner fire in the body (bronchitis, cough, pleurisy, phthisis, consumption).

The gum oozes from the incisions of natural fissures in the bark or the wood. It is cicatrizant and vulnerary and has powerful healing properties. It is especially useful in diseases related to secretion (inflammation of the breast or the uterus).

Putrefaction cannot take place in the desert; the air is too dry and the heat too intense. Burseraceae condense the desert energy and therefore have strong antiputrescent effects on corpses. They also have a salutary action

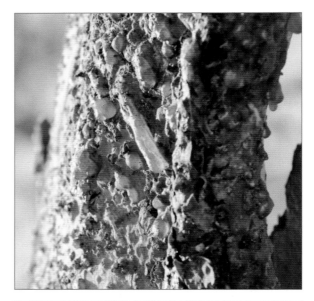

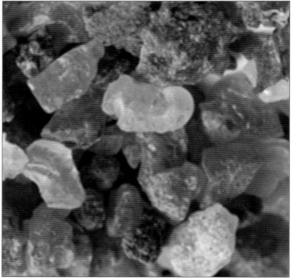

Myrrh gum exuding from tree bark (top); myrrh close-up (below)

on ulcers, gangrene, and gastric and intestinal fermentation.

The desert is also the place where those who want to go beyond the mundane and superfluous find an austere but powerful environ. There, everything is reduced to essentials. The contemplation of the endless petrified waves of the sandy dunes inspires one to go beyond the always-changing waves of one's own mind and connect with bare infinity and eternity. The powerful comforting scent of myrrh or frankincense carried by the burning wind of the desert gently soothes one's deepest wounds and gives one further inspiration in meditation.

Since antiquity, myrrh and frankincense have been extensively used in incense in rituals and religious ceremonies. They have a very pronounced soothing, comforting, fortifying, and elevating action on the soul and the spirit.

Type of action: Cooling, drying, fortifying
Domain of action: Skin, lungs, secretion, mind, psychic centers
Indications: Inflammation (skin, lungs, breast, uterus)

Elemi (*Canarium luzonicum*)

- Gum is primarily produced in the Philippines, Central America, and Brazil
- Essential oil is distilled from the gum; it is colorless to slightly yellow
- Fragrance: Pleasant, balsamic (resembling camphor), and incenselike
- Used in perfumery and in some medical preparations

Introduced to Europe in the fifteenth century, elemi was an ingredient in numerous balms, unguents, and liniments. It is still used in the balm of Fioraventi and other vulnerary preparations.

Medicinal properties and indications: Similar to those of myrrh and frankincense (see below)

Frankincense (*Boswellia carterii*)

- Gum is primarily produced in northeast Africa and southeast Arabia (Somalia, Ethiopia, Yemen); the supply has been quite erratic lately because of the political confusion in these countries
- Essential oil is distilled from the gum; it is clear or yellow
- Fragrance: Characteristic—balsamic, camphorlike, spicy, woody, and slightly lemony
- Used in cosmetics and perfumery; blends well with almost any scent; makes a good fixative

One of the most highly priced substances of the ancient world, frankincense was once as valuable as gold. Its trade was one of the major economic activities in some Arabic countries, and its control provoked many local wars. The Queen of Sheba, a main producer of that time, undertook a perilous journey from Somalia to Israel and visited King Solomon to secure the flourishing trade. Frankincense has been burned in temples since antiquity, especially by the Egyptians and the Hebrews; it is still used in the rites of some churches. Frankincense gum was traditionally used to fumigate sick persons to drive out the evil spirits causing the sickness. The Egyptians used it in their rejuvenating unguents.

Medicinal properties and indications: Similar to those of myrrh (see page 108); special action on breast inflammations and uterine disorders; pregnancy, childbirth preparation

Myrrh (*Commiphora myrrha*)

- Gum is primarily produced in the same areas as frankincense, as well as in Libya and Iran
- Essential oil is distilled from the gum; it is yellow to reddish brown and more or less fluid
- Fragrance: Pleasant, balsamic, camphorlike, musky, and incenselike
- Used in perfumery and cosmetics; blends well with many oils; makes a good fixative

The history of myrrh is closely tied to that of frankincense. These two substances were among the precious drugs reserved for fumigations, embalming, unctions, and liturgical practices. The Egyptian papyri, the Vedas, the Bible, and the Koran mention the numerous uses of myrrh in ceremonies, in perfumery, and in medicine. Myrrh was an ingredient of many unguents, elixirs, and other multipurpose antidotes.

Medicinal properties: Mucous fluidifier, expectorant; astringent, resolutive; anti-inflammatory, antiseptic, antiputrescent, vulnerary, cicatrizant; affects mucous membranes; stimulant, tonic; sedative

Indications: Inflammation (breast, lungs, gangrene, infected wounds, ulcers); catarrhal conditions (head, lungs, stomach, intestines); tuberculosis, phthisis, bronchitis, cough; hemorrhages (uterine, pulmonary); pregnancy, childbirth

CISTACEAE
The Rock Rose Family

Cistaceae are a small family of beautiful small shrubs that are profusely covered by flowers during the blooming season. They grow well in poor soils and prefer dry and sunny habitats. They are found in temperate or warm-temperate areas, especially the Mediterranean region. They have hard-coated, impermeable seeds that soften under heat, which makes them optimally adapted to repopulate areas destroyed by wildfires.

Many Cistaceae are fragrant and sweet-smelling. Various *Cistus* species secrete labdanum, a sticky exudate coating their leaves and stems, mostly in summer.

Cistus (*Cistus ladanifer*)

- Primarily produced in Spain and Cyprus
- Essential oil is distilled from the branches; it is reddish brown
- Fragrance: Musky and balsamic
- Used in expensive perfumes because it makes a good fixative and gives a natural musk note to the blends

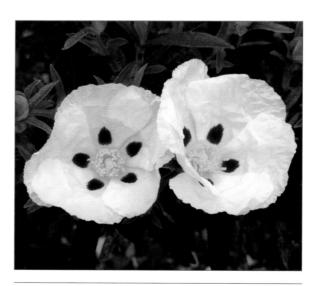

Cistus

Cistus, or rock rose, is a small bush growing in dry rocky areas of the Mediterranean countries, especially in Crete and Cyprus. Its leaves naturally exude a gum called labdanum. This gum has been highly appreciated in perfumery, cosmetics, and medicine since antiquity and was one of the ingredients of the "holy ointment" of the Bible.

The gum sticks to the wool of sheep grazing on the hills as they walk through the bushes, so shepherds in Crete and Cyprus used to comb the wool of their sheep to collect the precious gum. Labdanum was also collected by whipping the bushes with a special whip, this method giving a much better quality. Unfortunately both methods have now been abandoned, and labdanum is not produced anymore.

Medicinal properties: Tonic, astringent; nervous sedative, antispasmodic; vulnerary

Indications: Diarrhea, dysentery, intestinal troubles; nervousness, insomnia; ulcers

CONIFERAE (PINOPHYTA)
Light and Inner Warmth versus Cold and Verticality

The Coniferae (sometimes known as the Pinophyta or Coniferophyta) are a division of gymnosperms—that is, cone-bearing seed plants. They include three major families: Cupressaceae and Pinaceae, both discussed below, and Taxaceae, commonly known as the yew family, which does not produce essential oils.

A wide belt of Coniferae circles the frigid and temperate zones of both hemispheres, from the far north or far south and almost to the mountaintops, depending on altitude. In tropical zones they grow only at high altitudes.

The type is imposing in its simplicity and dominated by a vertical and linear principle. Everything is structured around the central vertical trunk; the trunk is surrounded with branches shaped like small trees, and the leaves are reduced to long needles placed in spirals around the twigs. The floral process is reduced to its minimum: the cone of flowers, a termi-

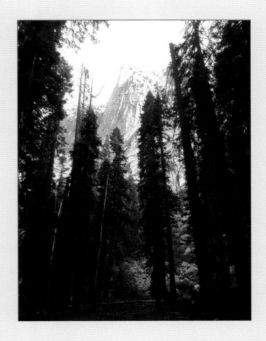

nal twig surrounded by dense ligneous leaves, bears the nude reproductive organs (stamens or pistil) on the axil of its leaves. The longevity of Coniferae, ruled by Saturn, gives us the oldest and highest trees in the world. In some species, the trunks themselves are virtually immune to rot (prehistoric cypresses found in coal mines in

Silesia were used to make furniture!). The coniferous forest appears immemorial and eternal. Its solemnity, noble majesty and powerful magnificence bring us back to primordial nature. This forest inspires devotion and respect and opens the heart "to the most ancient, the most basic and primordial feelings of the creation" (Goethe). Troubled souls find rest and strength here.

Coniferae also produce in abundance etheric oils and resins, which fill up the trunks, branches, and needles. In certain species the resin production is so intense that the trees exude it through their cones or their trunks. Such a phenomenon indicates a deep characteristic relationship between this type and the forces of light and warmth. Because Coniferae live in cold climates, they have to develop an intense inner fire to face the long, rigorous winters until the overflowing light of summer, with its clear nights and its midnight sun. These processes of warmth relate to life and generate substances (essential oils, resins, balms) that are at the origin of the curative power of Coniferae, which is warming and revivifying. Their zone of action is the cold area of the body: the nervous system. The oils of Coniferae are best taken through the lungs (inhalation or aromatic diffuser), where they communicate the prajna energy of the type.

Type of action: Tonic, revivifying, appeasing, warming

Domain of action: Nervous system, lungs, glandular system

Indications: Stress, deficiency of the nervous system, lung problems, rheumatism, arthritis

CUPRESSACEAE
Trees of Longevity

Essential oils of this family include cypress, juniper, and thuja. Other oils of interest are cade, fokienia, and savin juniper.

The Cupressaceae family counts 27 genera, including *Cupressus, Juniperus, Sequoia and sequoiadendron* (redwoods), *Thuja,* and *Calocedrus,* and 142 species. It is the most widely distributed of all gymnosperm families, being found on all continents except Antarctica.

Cupressaceae is a family of superlatives, with *Sequoiadendron giganteum,* the largest of all trees; *Sequoia sempervirens,* the tallest of all trees; and four of the five oldest known trees from nonclonal species on Earth, listed below.

Fitzroya cupressoides (oldest specimen: 3,622 years)

Sequoiadendron giganteum (oldest specimen: 3,266 years)

Juniperus grandis (oldest specimen: 2,675 years)

Taxodium distichum (oldest specimen: 2,624 years)

The heartwood of many species of Cupressaceae is resistant to termite damage and fungal decay, and therefore it is widely used for

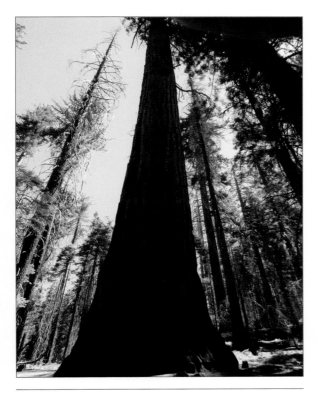

Sequoia

building where wood must be in contact with the elements, such as fenceposts, roofing shingles, siding, lawn furniture, and even coffins in China and Japan. Many genera are incorrectly called cedars because their heartwood is as aromatic as that of the true cedars, *Cedrus* spp. (of the Pinaceae family).

Many Cupressaceae are highly venerated by traditional societies. *Cryptomeria japonica* is the national tree of Japan, and four of the five sacred trees of Kiso belong to this family. *Thuja plicata* is highly revered among the tribes of the Northwest of North America. And sequoia and *Sequoiadendron* species inspire a deep sense of awe and wonder in all who see them.

Cypress (*Cupressus sempervirens*)

- Primarily produced in France, Spain, and Morocco
- Essential oil is distilled from the branches; it is yellow to brown
- Fragrance: Balsamic, woody, and somewhat harsh

The ancient Egyptians used cypress in their medical preparations; its wood, almost immune to rot, was used to make the sarcophagi for mummies.

Medicinal properties: Astringent, vasoconstrictor, tonic for the veins; antispasmodic; diuretic, antirheumatic, antisudorific; antiseptic

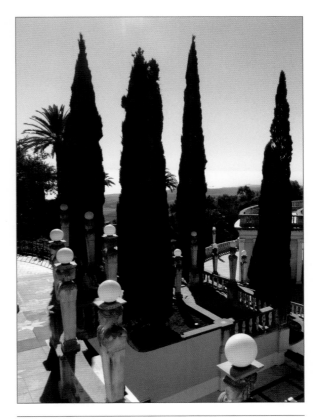

Cypress

Indications: Hemorrhoids, varicose veins; enuresis; whooping cough, asthma; ovary dysfunction (dysmenorrhea, menopausal problems); perspiration

Juniper (*Juniperus communis*)

- Primarily produced in Yugoslavia, Italy, and France
- Essential oil is distilled from the berries (gives the best quality) or the small branches; it is colorless, yellowish, or pale green
- Fragrance: Terebinthinate, hot, and balsamic

Juniper was burned as incense to ward off evil spirits or to serve as a disinfectant in times of epidemic diseases. Tibetans used it for religious and medicinal purposes. This smallest of the Coniferae grows in arid and inhospitable areas, where its presence is like a consolation. During Christmas ceremonies in Germany it represents the tree of life. It hides its rough, bitter fruits in the midst of thick needles; these fruits are salutary for everyone who has abused terrestrial food. It is an excellent diuretic, digestive, and hepatic. Its distorted shape and hard, knotty, twisted wood indicate an obvious affinity with joints, arthritis, and rheumatism. Juniper can influence the effects of old age.

Medicinal properties: Diuretic, antiseptic (urinary tract), antirheumatic (promotes the elimination of uric acid and toxins); stomachic; antidiabetic; tonic (nervous system, visceral functions, digestive system); fortifies the memory; rubefacient; vulnerary

Indications: Urinary tract infections, kidney stones, blennorrhea, cystitis, oliguria; diabetes; rheumatism, arteriosclerosis; general weariness, nervous fatigue; amenorrhea, dysmenorrhea, painful menstruation; dermatitis, eczema

Thuja (*Thuja occidentalis*)

- Primarily produced in Canada and the United States (Vermont, New Hampshire).
- Essential oil is distilled from the small branches and twigs; it is yellowish.
- Essential oil is highly toxic; it should not be taken internally without the supervision of a medical specialist.

Medicinal properties: Diuretic, urinary sedative; expectorant; antirheumatic; vermifuge
Indications: Prostatic hypertrophy, cystitis; rheumatism; intestinal parasites; warts

PINACEAE
Air and Inner Fire

Essential oils of this family include cedarwood, fir, pine, and spruce. Other oils of interest are hemlock (*Tsuga canadensis*) and terebinth.

With 10 genera and 250 species of shrubs and trees, the Pinaceae family is the largest, most widespread and abundant conifer family in the Northern Hemisphere, often being the dominant component of boreal, coastal, and montane forests. It includes many conifers of important economic value such as cedars, firs, hemlocks, larches, pines, and spruces.

The bristlecone pine (*Pinus longaeva*) known as Methusaleh in Nevada is 4,851 years old and the oldest known living nonclonal organism on Earth.

To protect themselves against antagonists,

Pinaceae have evolved numerous mechanical and/or chemical defenses, mostly prevalent in the bark of the trees as resins, phenolics, and polyphenols. The resins also help make them resistant to extreme temperatures.

Cedarwood (*Cedrus atlantica*)

- Primarily produced in Morocco
- The essential oil is distilled from the sawdust; it is is thick and golden brown, like the color of old gold
- Fragrance: Deep, woody, balsamic, and very pleasant; like sandalwood

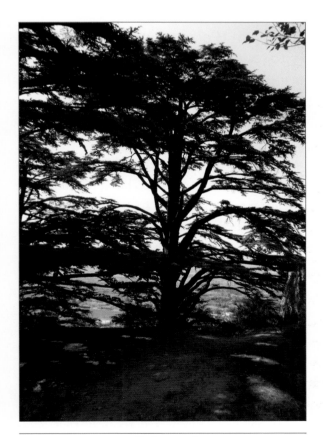

Cedarwood

- Used as a fixative in perfumes; blends well with many oils and gives a woody note to preparations

The Himalayan cedar (*Cedrus deodorata*) is distilled in the Himalayas. The Eastern red cedar, distilled in the United States, is actually a juniper (*Juniperus virginiana*); its essential oil, however, is very similar to real cedarwood essential oil.

Egyptians used cedarwood oil for embalming; it was one of the ingredients of *mithridat,* a famous poison antidote that was used for centuries. One of the most majestic trees, the Lebanese cedar (like its close relative, atlas cedar, growing in Morocco) expresses a great spiritual strength. Egyptians used its wood to build the doors of their temples, where its fragrance would stimulate psychic centers of the worshipers. The effects of cedarwood oil on the mind are similar to those of sandalwood.

Medicinal properties: Antiseptic, fungicidal, antiputrescent; expectorant; stimulant
Indications: Cystitis, gonorrhea, urinary tract disorders; hair care (hair loss, dandruff, scalp diseases); respiratory conditions; skin disease (eczema, dermatitis, ulcers); anxiety, nervous tension

Fir (*Abies balsamea*)

- Primarily produced in the northeast United States and Canada
- Essential oil is distilled from the branches; it is colorless
- Fragrance: Fresh, balsamic, and very pleasant; one of the finest coniferous scents

The fir tree exudes a resin called fir balsam that the North American Indians used for medicinal and religious purposes. It was introduced to Europe in the beginning of the seventeenth century, and its action was compared to that of Venetian turpentine, which was highly valued at the time.

Medicinal properties: Respiratory antiseptic, expectorant; vulnerary
Indications: Respiratory diseases; genitourinary infections

Pine (*Pinus sylvestris*)

🌿 Produced all over the world
🌿 Essential oil is distilled from the small branches; it is colorless

Various species closely related to *P. sylvestris* are distilled in Austria, Italy, and Yugoslavia. Primarily produced in the former Soviet Union, Germany, and France, *P. maritimus* is distilled in France.

Medicinal properties: Expectorant, pulmonary antiseptic; stimulant of adrenocortical glands; hepatic and urinary antiseptic; rubefacient
Indications: Pulmonary diseases; urinary infections

Spruce (*Picea mariana*)

🌿 Produced in the same area as fir
🌿 Essential oil is distilled from the branches; it is colorless
🌿 Fragrance: Similar to fir, but deeper

Spruce oil is excellent for balancing energy. It is recommended for any type of psychic work for its opening and elevating, though grounding, quality. In a diffuser it is excellent for yoga and meditation.

Medicinal properties and indications: Same as for fir

GERANIACEAE
Chameleons of the Fragrant Realm

Geraniaceae are flowering herbs or subshrubs widely used in gardening. The family includes both true geraniums and pelargoniums, native to South Africa, which produce highly valued essential oils.

Geranium (*Pelargonium graveolens, P. roseum*)

🌿 Primarily produced in Réunion, Comoro Islands, Egypt, and Morocco
🌿 Essential oil is distilled from the whole plant; it is greenish yellow
🌿 Fragrance: Strong, sweet, and roselike (almost too strong when it is pure, but it becomes very pleasant when diluted)
🌿 Widely used in perfumery and cosmetics; blends very well with rose, citrus, and almost any oil

Old herbals mention the geranium called herb Robert (*Geranium robertianum*), which grows wild in the temperate zones of the globe. This plant is totally different from the pelargonium used for the extraction of essential oils. Although the two species belong to the same botanical family, their uses are different.

It has been discovered recently that geranium has the power to develop an extremely

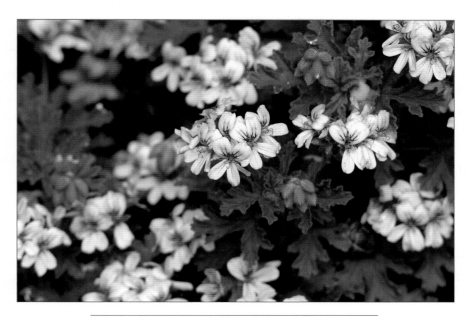

Geranium

wide variety of chemotypes, none of them being distilled commercially at this point. The reason for such variations is not yet clear. In fact, geranium can be made to imitate almost any fragrance. In addition to the rose geranium, others—tangerine geranium, lemon geranium, lime geranium, and the like—are found in nurseries. Apparently the species can produce almost any possible chemotype, including those with the hot, burning thymols and carvacrols that seem so remote from the sweet-smelling rose geranium that most people know. This seems to indicate a strong adaptability, indicative of immunostimulant properties.

Related organ: Kidneys
Medicinal properties: Astringent, hemostatic, cicatrizant, antiseptic; antidiabetic, diuretic; stimulant of adrenal cortex; insect repellent

Indications: Diabetes, kidney stones; adrenocortical deficiency; tonsillitis, sore throat; hemorrhage; burns, wounds, ulcers; skin disease, skin care; nervous tension, depression

LAMIACEAE (LABIATAE)
Plants of Heat; the Healing Family

Essential oils of this family include basil, hyssop, lavender, lavandin, marjoram, melissa, mints (pennyroyal, peppermint, spearmint), oregano, patchouli, rosemary, sage, spike lavender, and thyme. While medicinal plants are the exception in most families, all Lamiaceae have some curative power, which indicates their special relationship to humans. This phenomenon is due to the extraordinary influence of the cosmic forces of heat on the formation of the family. This calorific nature leads to the formation of essential oils.

Lamiaceae have special predilection for open spaces, dry and rocky slopes, and sunny mountains, where their most characteristic species (lavender, rosemary, sage, thyme) appear. They prefer median climatic regions all around the Mediterranean and far from tropical and cold areas. Many Lamiaceae are culinary herbs, which indicates their affinity for the digestive processes. Their fragrance is invigorating, stimulating, fiery, and reawakening. There are no bland, gloomy, ecstatic, or narcotic notes in this family.

Finally, many Lamiaceae (including basil, peppermint, rosemary, and thyme) have the power to develop chemotypes. This seems to indicate a strong potential for adaptability in the family, which could be interpreted as immunostimulant power. (Geranium is another plant with many chemotypes, and it is also considered an immunostimulant.)

Type of action: Warming, stimulating (vital center, metabolism); appeasing effect on overactive astral body; brings it back under the control of vital centers

Domain of action: Organization of vital centers—metabolism, digestion, respiration, blood formation

Indications: Weakness of vital centers (anemia, poor digestion, respiratory problems, diabetes); recommended for people with intense psychic activity (healers, mediums, etc.) to keep them from losing control and depleting their vitality

Basil (*Ocimum basilicum*)

🍃 Primarily produced in India, Egypt, Comoro Islands, and Réunion

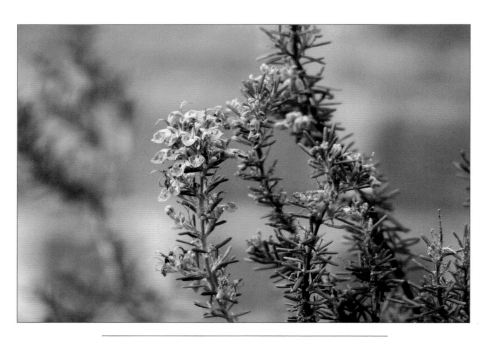

Rosemary in flower

- Essential oil is distilled from the herb; it is yellow
- Fragrance: Pleasant and anise-y, with a minty note
- Used in perfumery for its top green note; blends well with bergamot or geranium

There are several chemotypes of basil (there is even a cinnamon basil); the most commonly used is the methychavicol type (from Réunion and the Comoro Islands), as well as the eugenol type. One of the sacred plants of India, where it is dedicated to Vishnu, basil is extensively used in Ayurvedic medicine. Its actions on the digestive and nervous systems have been acknowledged in both Indian and Western medicine.

Related organs: Neurovegetative and digestive systems
Medicinal properties: Nervous tonic, antispasmodic, cephalic; stomachic, intestinal antiseptic; stupefying at high doses
Indications: Mental fatigue, migraine, insomnia, depression, mental strain; dyspepsia, gastric spasms; intestinal infections; facilitates childbirth and nursing

Hyssop (*Hyssopus officinalis*)

- Primarily produced in France, Spain, and southern Europe
- Essential oil is distilled from the whole plant in flower; it is golden yellow
- Fragrance: Nicely aromatic; reminiscent of sage, marjoram, and lavender

One of the sacred plants of the Hebrews, hyssop (*esobh*) was prescribed by Hippocrates, Galen, and Dioscorides for its curative power on the respiratory system. The ancient pharmacopoeia mentions it as the major ingredient in numerous preparations, elixirs, and syrups.

Hyssop grows all over southern Europe and western Asia on dry, rocky slopes, but its finest varieties grow above 3,000 feet in the sunny meadows of the southern Alps. Its abundant leaf system and its camphorlike scent indicate its special affinity for the respiratory system.

Related organ: Lungs
Medicinal properties: Expectorant (liquefies bronchial secretions), antitussive, emollient; antispasmodic; tonic (especially for the heart and respiration); hypertensive agent, regulates blood pressure; digestive, stomachic; sudorific, febrifuge; cicatrizant, vulnerary
Indications: Hypotension; respiratory diseases (asthma, bronchitis, catarrh, cough, tuberculosis); poor digestion, dyspepsia, flatulence; dermatitis, eczema, wounds; syphilis; urinary stones

Lavender (*Lavandula officinalis*)

- One of the most precious essential oils
- Primarily produced in France, Spain, and countries of the former Soviet Union
- Essential oil is distilled from the flowers; it is clear to yellowish green
- Fragrance: Clean, classic, and appeasing
- Best variety is called "fine lavender"; others include Maillette and Materonne

Lavender was a favorite aromatic used by the Romans in their baths (the word comes from the Latin *lavare*). Dioscorides, Pliny, and Galen

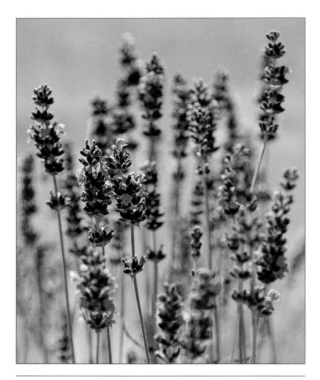

Lavender

mention it as a stimulant, tonic, stomachic, and carminative. It has always been used in perfumery and cosmetics and blends well with a great number of essential oils, adding a light floral note to almost any preparation.

Far from the ardor of rosemary, lavender emanates a noble, mellow peacefulness. Its blue flowers bloom at the top of a structure resembling a seven-branched candlestick; they give a clean, soothing scent that is one of our most beautiful perfumes.

The finest quality of lavender grows above 3,000 feet on the sunny slopes of the southern Alps and up to the mountaintops. Lavender likes air, space, light, and warmth. It has an appeasing action on the astral body; it tones and soothes the nervous system and is beneficial for the respiratory system.

Medicinal properties: Calming, analgesic, antispasmodic, anticonvulsive, antidepressant; antiseptic, healing; cytophylactic; diuretic, antirheumatic; insect repellent

Indications: Respiratory diseases (asthma, bronchitis, catarrh, influenza, whooping cough, throat infections); sinusitis; migraine, depression, convulsions, nervous tension, fainting, insomnia, neurasthenia, palpitations; infectious diseases; skin diseases: abscess, acne dermatitis. eczema, pediculosis, psoriasis; burns, wounds; leukorrhea; cystitis, mucus discharge; insect bites

Lavandin (*Lavandula fragrans, L. delphinensis*)

The lavandins are hybrids of true lavender and spike; their essential oils have a lower ester content and contain some camphor. Their fragrance is not as refined as that of lavender; their medicinal properties are similar, though less potent.

Main varieties: The finest are Super and Abrialis; Grosso is also worth considering

Veterinary uses: Antiseptic, vulnerary, dermatitis, scabies

Spike (*Lavandula spica*)

Spike lavender grows below 2,000 feet. Its essential oils contain some camphor; it calms the cerebrospinal activity. It is also used as an insecticide and for veterinary purposes.

Marjoram (*Origanum marjorana, Marjorana hortensis*)

- Other variety: Wild spanish marjoram (*Thymus mastichina*)
- Primarily produced in Spain (wild Spanish marjoram), Egypt, North Africa, and Hungary
- Essential oil is distilled from the plant in flower; it is colorless to yellowish
- Fragrance: Sweet and appeasing; one of the nicest of Lamiaceae oils
- Used in perfumery and cosmetics; blends well with lavender and bergamot

Marjoram was grown in ancient Egypt, and Greeks and Romans used it to weave crowns for the newly married. According to mythology, Aphrodite, goddess of love and fecundity, picked marjoram on Mount Ida to heal the wounds of Enea. According to Dioscorides, it tones and warms the nerves; Pliny recommends it for poor digestion and a weak stomach; and Culpeper praises its warming and comforting effects.

Rather than altitude and rocks, marjoram prefers the light warm soil of gardens. The plant is sweet looking and delicate, with small, round, soft, velvety leaves and cute little white flowers, almost hidden among the leaves. Its gentle and appeasing fragrance has a warming and comforting effect, hence its beneficent action on the nervous system. Marjoram also has a warming action on the metabolism and genital organs.

Related organs: Peripheral nervous system
Medicinal properties: Antispasmodic, calming, sedative, analgesic, anaphrodisiac; hypotensive, arterial vasodilator; digestive; narcotic in high doses
Indications: Spasms (digestive, pulmonary), insomnia, migraine, nervous tension, neurasthenia, anxiety; hypertension; dyspepsia, flatulence; arthritis, rheumatic pain

Melissa (*Melissa officinalis*)

- Primarily produced in France
- Essential oil is distilled from the whole plant; it is colorless to yellowish
- Fragrance: Fresh, lemony, and very pleasant

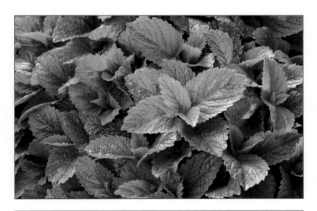

Melissa

Melissa (sometimes called balm or lemon balm, or *citronelle* in French) has a very low yield (about 0.05 percent) of essential oil. The production of the oil had been virtually abandoned until the late 1980s, when a few French producers started distilling it again. It is a very expensive essential oil and is therefore widely adulterated (the most common additives are lemongrass, citronella, and *Litsea cubeba*). So-called melissa oil has been sold, especially in England, at a fraction of the production cost of true melissa oil. While total world production of melissa essential oil was less than 50 pounds in 1988, total sales worldwide could have been well over 1,000 pounds (another miracle of modern technology)! Patricia Davis, in her excellent *Aromatherapy: An A–Z,* warns against possible skin irritations when using melissa essential oil externally. One wonders whether she used true melissa oil in the first place, since most of what is available for purchase is adulterated.

The plant is named after the Greek nymph Melissa, protectress of the bees. In spring, when several queens are born in the same beehive, the swarm splits into several smaller swarms, and each has to look for a new hive. Fresh melissa leaves were traditionally crushed on empty hives to attract the migrant swarms.

Melissa is a gentle and humble-looking plant with pale green leaves and small white to light pink flowers. There emanates from the whole plant a natural kindness that is soothing and comforting in itself. Melissa was traditionally considered calming and uplifting; it is soothing, relieves tension, and is, with rose and neroli, one of the major oils for the heart chakra.

Melissa seems to thrive on iron. It likes the vicinity of houses, especially in the country where nails and other pieces of scrap iron are often buried around habitations. When I was a wildcrafter, the place where I could find the most abundant crop of melissa was an abandoned iron mine. This indicates a possible antianemic and immunostimulant property; indeed, melissa has been known to strengthen vitality.

Medicinal properties: Antispasmodic, calming, sedative, soothing; antidepressant, uplifting; digestive; antiviral; stimulant of the heart chakra

Indications: Insomnia; migraine, nervous tension, neurasthenia, anxiety; cold sores, shingles; emotional shock, grief

Mints: Pennyroyal, Peppermint, Spearmint

Pluto once fell in love with the nymph Mintha, but his wife, the jealous Proserpine, changed her into the plant that is now named after her. According to Pliny, "The scent of mint awakens the mind and its taste excites the appetite and the stomach." Its fortifying and stimulating qualities have been acknowledged by Roman and Greek physicians.

There are about twenty species in the genus *Mentha,* growing all over the world. They like abundant light and deep, humid soils. In them, the warmth principle struggles against an adverse principle of cold and water, and hence these herbs have a warming, stimulating, curative power good for resolving congestion, cramps, and swelling; promote menstruation; and stimulate virility. On the other hand, mints also have vivifying, refreshing, and appeasing qualities.

Common medicinal properties of the genus Mentha: Nervous system stimulant, general tonic, antispasmodic; stomachic, digestive, carminative; hepatic, cholagogue; expectorant; emmenagogue; febrifuge; antiseptic

Indications: Gastralgia, dyspepsia, nausea, flatulence, vomiting; mental fatigue, migraine, headache, fainting, neuralgia; dysmenorrhea; hepatic disorders; cold, cough, asthma, bronchitis; neuralgia

Pennyroyal (*Mentha pulegium*)

- Primarily produced in Spain and North Africa
- Essential oil is distilled from the whole plant; it is colorless to yellowish
- Fragrance: Resembles peppermint, but harsher

Specific medicinal properties and indications: Amenorrhea (warning: pennyroyal is abortive at high doses); splenetic

Peppermint (*Mentha piperita*)

- Produced all over the world, the United States being the biggest producer; the finest quality comes from England and southern France
- Essential oil is distilled from the whole plant; it is colorless
- Numerous uses in perfumery, cosmetics, and food industry (liquors, sauces, drinks, candies, etc.)

Mentha piperita has several subspecies and chemotypes (*M. piperita* var. *bergamia, M. piperita* chemotype linalool, etc.), none of them being commercially distilled as far as I know.

Specific indications: Impotence

Spearmint (*Mentha viridis*)

The fragrance of spearmint is very similar to that of peppermint but is fresher and less harsh. Its therapeutic activity is approximately the same.

Oregano (*Origanum vulgare, O. compactum, Coridothymus capitatus*)

- Primarily produced in Spain, North Africa, and Greece (many subspecies)
- Essential oil is distilled from the herb; it is brownish red
- Fragrance: Burning, spicy, and strongly aromatic

Although the ancients often grouped different species under this name, oregano had been considered an essential aromatic plant for medicine and for cooking since antiquity. Theophrastes, Aristotle, and Hippocrates praised its beneficent action on respiratory diseases, ulcers, burns, and poor digestion.

A rustic variant of marjoram, oregano grows wild all over Europe and Asia; however, only the Mediterranean varieties yield a significant amount of essential oils. Their hot, almost burning quality indicates their beneficent action on infectious diseases, infected wounds, and inflammations.

Medicinal properties: Antiseptic, antitoxic, antivirus; antispasmodic, sedative; expectorant; analgesic, counterirritant
Indications: Infectious diseases, disinfection; bronchopulmonary diseases; rheumatism; pediculosis; amenorrhea

Patchouli (*Pogostemon patchouli*)

- Primarily produced in India, Malaysia, Burma, and Paraguay
- Essential oil is distilled from the dried,

fermented leaves; it is thick and brown to greenish brown

🍃 Fragrance: Strong, sweet, musky, and very persistent

🍃 Used in dermatology, aesthetics, and skin care. One of the best fixatives, used in small amounts in Eastern and rose perfumes

Patchouli essential oil was part of the materia medica in Malaysia, China, India, and Japan, where it was used for its stimulant, tonic, stomachic, and febrifuge properties. It was a renowned antidote against insect and snake bites. Indians also used it to scent their fabrics, especially the famous Indian shawls so fashionable in England in the nineteenth century. The essential oil contains patchoulene and other products close to azulene.

One of the most tropical Lamiaceae, patchouli is a plant of excessive warmth and water; its large leaves and its morphology indicate that these energies are not fully dominated. Therefore, although it is a stimulant and tonic at low doses, good for dissipating the type of lethargy related to such energies (sluggishness, inertia), it becomes sedative or even stupefying at high doses. Its anti-inflammatory and decongestive properties also derive from these characteristics. Because the essential oil is produced after a period of fermentation, it has certain control over all processes of stagnation, putrefaction, and aging (uses in skin care and rejuvenation). *Opus niger* (black work), which in the physical world is a process of fermentation and putrefaction, is one of the major phases of the alchemist's work, a phase conducive to the illu-

mination of the adept after cold burning of all impurities and decantation. Patchouli is then a product of fermentation in the alchemical sense. It has powerful action on the psychic centers on a metaphysical level.

Medicinal properties: Decongestive, antiphlogistic, anti-inflammatory, tissue regenerator, fungicide, anti-infectious, bactericidal; stimulant (nervous system) at low doses; sedative at high doses; rejuvenating to the skin; insect repellent

Indications: Mucous discharge, sluggishness; skin care (seborrhea, eczema, dermatitis, impetigo, herpes, cracked skin, wrinkles); anxiety, depression; insect and snake bites

Rosemary (*Rosmarinus officinalis*)

🍃 Produced all around the Mediterranean Sea

🍃 Essential oil is distilled from the herb; it is almost colorless

🍃 Fragrance: Fiery, aromatic, and invigorating, with a dominant note reminiscent of eucalyptus (for the Spanish and North African varieties) and of frankincense (more pronounced in the French and Yugoslavian varieties)

Like thyme, but to a lesser degree, rosemary has developed several chemotypes, growing in fairly distinct climatic areas. The phenol-cineole chemotype grows in North Africa (Morocco and Tunisia), the cineole chemotype grows in Spain, and the verbenon chemotype grows in southern France, Corsica, northern Italy, and Yugoslavia.

This vigorous, thick bush has a predilection for rocky, sunny slopes and grows all around the Mediterranean, from the seashore to about 2,000 feet. It has been used extensively since antiquity for medicine and in cooking as well as for rituals. Highly praised in the Middle Ages and the Renaissance, it appeared in various formulas such as the famous Queen of Hungary's water, a rejuvenating liquor. (At the age of seventy-two, when she was gouty and paralytic, Elizabeth of Hungary received the recipe from an angel, or a monk, and recovered her health and beauty.) Madame de Sevigny recommended rosemary water for sadness.

A calorific plant above all, rosemary, according to Rudolf Steiner, fortifies the vital center and its action of other constituents of the human being. It restores the balance of the calorific body and activates the blood processes (blood is the privileged medium of the healing principle in the human body). It is thus recommended for anemia, insufficient menstruation, and troubles of blood irrigation. Its acts on the liver as well.

A better irrigation of the organs eases the action of astral and vital forces and stimulates metabolism. Thus rosemary is digestive and sudorific; it promotes the assimilation of sugar (in diabetes) and is indicated to rebuild the nervous system after long, intense intellectual activity.

Related organs: Liver, gallbladder
Medicinal properties: General stimulant, cardiotonic, stimulant of adrenocortical glands; cholagogue, hepatobiliary stimulant (increases biliary secretion); pulmonary antiseptic; diuretic, sudorific; antirheumatismal, antineuralgic, rubefacient; healing for wounds and burns
Indications: Hepatobiliary disorders (cholecystitis, cirrhosis, gallstone, hypercholesterolaemia, jaundice); general weakness, anemia, asthenia, debility, menstruation; mental fatigue, mental strain, loss of memory; colds, bronchitis, whooping cough; rheumatism, gout; hair loss, dandruff; skin care; wounds, burns; scabies, pediculosis

Salvia

With more than five hundred species, the genus *Salvia* is the most important of the Lamiaceae family. *Salvia officinalis* likes chalky rocks and the desert mountains of Spain, Greece, Dalmatia, and the Balkans. Its fragrance is severe, solemn, earthy, and harsh. Its well-developed leaves and large, odoriferous flowers shaped to receive the bodies of bees indicate its affinity for all processes of life and creation—even procreation. *S. sclarea* (clary sage) goes even

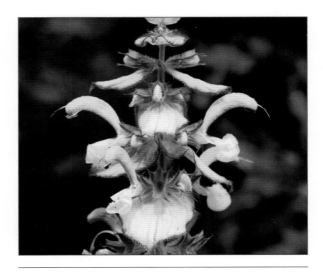

Clary sage

further; reduced for years to a few small leaves close to the ground, it suddenly develops wide, thick leaves and extravagant flowers atop high, square stems, suggesting the quiet confidence and radiance of a pregnant woman. It was preeminently the plant of women in their creative process and was particularly indicated to induce and promote pregnancy.

Clary Sage (*Salvia sclarea*)

- Primarily produced in southern France, countries of the former Soviet Union, and the United States
- Essential oil is distilled from the whole plant; it is clear
- Fragrance: Pleasant, sweet with floral notes, and slightly musky
- Widely used as a fixative in cosmetics and perfumery

Clary sage is preferred to other sages for long cures (with no toxicity).

Related organs: Female reproductive system
Medicinal properties and indications: Similar to those of *S. officinalis,* with a special emphasis on women's complaints pertaining to menstruation, leukorrhea, and frigidity

Sage (*Salvia officinalis*)

- Primarily produced in Spain, Yugoslavia, and France
- Essential oil is distilled from the leaves and flowers; it is colorless to yellowish
- Fragrance: Harsh and aromatic
- Sage essential oil is toxic at high doses and should not be taken internally for very long. It is not recommended for people with epileptic tendencies.

Renowned since antiquity, the *salvia salvatrix* of the Romans is one of the most powerful and versatile medicinal plants. Indeed, as they said, *Cur moriatur homo, cui salvia crescit in horto?* (Why should he die, the one who grows sage in his garden?) That panacea, which preserves health and youth, was always recommended for conception and pregnancy.

Related organs: Liver, gallbladder, kidneys
Medicinal properties: Toxic, stimulant (adrenocortical glands, nerves); antisudorific; antiseptic; diuretic; emmenagogue; hypertensive agent; aperitive, stomachic; depurative; astringent, vulnerary
Indications: General weakness, anemia, asthenia, neurasthenia; hypotension; sterility, menopause, regulation of menstruation, birth preparation; perspiration, fever; hepatobiliary and kidney dysfunctions; nervous afflictions; bronchitis, asthma; mouth ulcers, stomatitis, tonsillitis, dermatitis; hair loss; wounds, ulcers

Spanish Sage (*Salvia lavandulifolia*)

- Primarily produced in Spain
- Essential oil is distilled from the leaves and flowers; it is colorless to yellowish
- Fragrance: Finer and milder than *S. officinalis*

The therapeutic activity of *Salvia lavandulifolia* is similar to *S. Oficinalis,* but with low toxicity.

Thyme (*Thymus vulgaris*)

- Primarily produced in Morocco, Spain, France, and Greece
- Essential oil is distilled from the branches and flowers; it is red or brownish red for the thymol-carvacrol chemotypes and clear to yellowish for the other chemotypes
- Fragrance: Hot, spicy, and aromatic for the thymol-carvacrol chemotypes; sweet to fresh and green for the others (citrusy for the citral chemotype, roselike for the geraniol, etc.)

The genus *Thymus* produces many species, subspecies, and chemotypes all around the Mediterranean Sea (see appendix 1). It has been suggested that such variations may be caused by climatic and other environmental conditions. Thus the burning hot thymol and carvacrol chemotypes would grow at lower altitudes and in dryer climates, while the milder geraniol, linalool, citral, and thuyanol chemotypes would grow at higher altitudes and milder climates. It has even been suggested that a plant of thyme transplanted from one climatic area to another may begin to develop the characteristics of its new location (i.e., thyme growing in dryness at sea level would be a thymol-carvacrol chemotype, but it would become a linalool or geraniol chemotype if transplanted to a high altitude).

As seductive as this theory might be, the reality is slightly different. There is, in the wild, a predominance of the thymol and carvacrol chemotypes in the dryer and warmer areas, while the milder chemotypes are more abundant under milder conditions. But more than seven years of wild harvesting of thyme have shown me that the different chemotypes can be found everywhere. Furthermore, most of the commercial production of chemotyped thyme comes from the same area of southern France, and several farmers grow all the chemotypes on their farms.

This tiny bush, with no special requirements for soil quality or the amount of humidity, is quite avid for warmth and light. It is helpful whenever inner warmth is poor or missing: excess of water, chilling tendencies, cold, and weakness of the vital center, especially when it is manifested at the level of the lungs or stomach.

Thyme has been widely used for therapy since antiquity for its warming, stimulant, and cleansing properties. Thyme is able to create, by itself, almost the entire spectrum of fragrances demonstrated by the medicinal Lamiaceae family, from the burning thymol-carvacrol (reminiscent of oregano or savory) to the citral types (similar to melissa) and through the linalool types (akin to marjoram and lavender). This shows the amazing adaptability of the genus, its broad-spectrum curative power, and its incredible vital energy. Thymes certainly are among the major oils of aromatherapy.

Medicinal properties: General stimulant (physical, psychic, capillary circulation); antiseptic (lungs, intestines, genitourinary system); rubefacient; healing; mucous fluidifier, expectorant

Indications: Asthenia, anemia, neurasthenia, nervous deficiency; infectious diseases (intestinal and urinary); pulmonary diseases (bronchitis, tuberculosis, asthma); poor digestion, fermentation; rheumatism, arthritis, gout; flu, influenza, sore throat; wounds

LAURACEAE
Intense Etheric Activity

Lauraceae are mostly evergreen trees or shrubs with worldwide distribution in tropical and warm climates that are important components of tropical forests. Most of the species are strongly aromatic, indicative of intense etheric activity, with high concentrations of essential oils in their leaves, wood, and bark, which they use to repel parasites and predators. The wood of the camphor tree (*Cinnamomum camphora*), for instance, may be up to 5 percent crude essential oil, and a single tree can yield up to 3 tons of the oil.

The Lauraceae are often used as spices or for medicinal purposes. Their fragrant wood is prized for making insect-repellent furniture. Many species, most notoriously rosewood (*Aniba rosaeodora*), have been overexploited for timber or essential oil and are now endangered.

Their fruits are drupes that may be edible or produce vegetable oils. Avocado (*Persea americana*), for example, produces a highly nutritious fruit that is low in sugar and rich in protein, fat, and vitamins such as A, B, C, D, and E.

Essential oils of this family include cinnamon (both the bark and the leaves), *Litsea cubeba,* and rosewood. Other oils of interest are camphor, cassia, *Laurus nobilis,* ravensara, and sassafras.

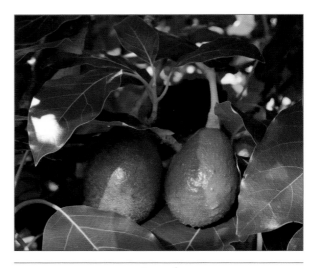

Avocado

Cinnamon (*Cinnamomum zeylanicum*)

- Primarily produced in Ceylon (the best quality), India, and China
- Essential oil is distilled from the bark; it is reddish brown
- Essential oil is also distilled from the leaves but is much lower quality
- Fragrance: Characteristically spicy and burning
- Widely used in the food industry, pharmacy, cosmetics, perfumery

Certainly one of the oldest spices known, cinnamon was already the object of an important trade between India, China, and Egypt more than four thousand years ago. In 2700 BC the Chinese emperor Shen Nung included it in his pharmacopoeia, calling it *kwei*. Cinnamon is often mentioned in the Bible. Yahweh ordered Moses to use it in the fabrication of the holy ointment. It was one of the most important drugs of the Greek and Roman pharmacopoeia and was quite renowned for its stomachic, diuretic, tonic, and antiseptic properties.

Medicinal properties: Stimulant (circulatory, cardiac, and pulmonary functions); antiseptic, antiputrescent; antispasmodic; aphrodisiac; parasiticide; irritant and convulsive in high doses
Indications: Flu, asthenia; spasms, intestinal infections; impotence; childbirth, labor (increases contractions)

May Chang (*Litsea cubeba*)

* Primarily produced in China
* Essential oil is distilled from the leaves; it is yellow
* Fragrance: Fresh, green, and lemony
* Widely used in perfumery and in the soap industry, deodorizers, sanitary products

Although its fragrance is closely related to that of citronella and lemongrass, *Litsea cubeba* has a much nicer scent. It is mostly used for blending (especially in the diffuser). It gives a pleasant, fresh, lemony top note to any blend.

Medicinal properties: Stimulant of the digestive system (stomachic, carminative, digestive); antiseptic; diuretic; insect repellent
Indications: Digestive troubles (dyspepsia, colic, flatulence); for disinfection or deodorization

Rosewood (*Aniba rosaeodora*)

* Primarily produced in Brazil
* Essential oil is distilled from the chopped wood; it is clear to pale yellow

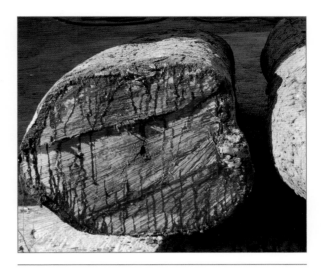

Rosewood

* Fragrance: Very sweet, floral, and woody
* Blends very well with almost any other essential oil

Rosewood essential oil is one of the major oils of perfumery, where it is used as a middle note. It was little used in aromatherapy until recently. Although it does not have any dramatic curative power (like tea tree or lavender), I find it very useful, especially for skin care. It is mild and safe to use. It is also very useful in blending; it helps give body to a blend and rounds out sharp edges. Rosewood is excellent for any type of body care or skin care preparation (bath oils, lotions, masks, facials).

Medicinal properties: Cellular stimulant, tissue regenerator; uplifting, antidepressant, tonic; calming, cephalic
Indications: Headache, nausea; skin care (sensitive skin, aged skin, wrinkles, general skin care); scars, wounds

MYRISTICACEAE
Intense Astral Activity

The evergreen flowering trees, shrubs, and, rarely, lianas of the Myristicaceae, or nutmeg, family are found in tropical rain forests across the world (humid lowland, swamps, and cloud forests). Most of the species are large trees valued for their timber.

Most species have fragrant wood and leaves. The small, highly reduced, fragrant flowers are either male or female and produce a starchy seed surrounded by a fleshy covering, known as an aril.

The family exhibits highly complex phyto-chemistry, with essential oils, alkaloids, and other compounds found in the leaves, bark, fruits, arils, and seeds of many species. The seeds of *Virola guatemalensis* are used in flavoring and in the manufacture of candles; the leaves are generally spicy and aromatic.

The tree bark in some genera, such as *Virola,* exudes a dark-red resin that contains several hallucinogenic alkaloids, indicative of intense astral activity. The bark of *Virola elongata* and other closely related species contains a derivative of tryptamine and is used by some Amazon tribes as a hallucinogenic snuff. Myristicin, found in nutmeg and its essential oil, is a strong deliriant that can induce convulsions, palpitations, and nausea; fatal myristicin poisonings have been reported.

Essential oils of this family include nutmeg. Another other oil of interest is mace.

Nutmeg (*Myristica fragrans*)

- Primarily produced in the West Indies, Indonesia, and Java
- Essential oil is distilled from the nuts; it is colorless
- The nut is surrounded by a fleshy shell, which, by distillation, yields an essential oil called mace oil; it is of lower quality than nutmeg oil, with similar composition and properties
- Fragrance: Spicy, peppery, and aromatic
- Some applications in pharmaceutical preparations; few uses in perfumery; widely used for the manufacture of spirits and elixirs

First mentioned in the fifth century, nutmeg was introduced to the West by Arabian

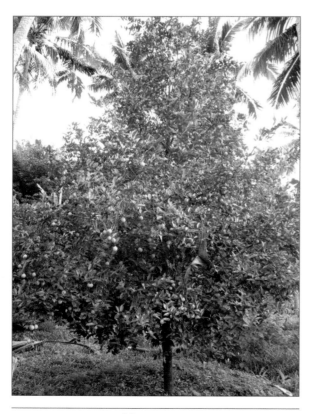

Nutmeg tree

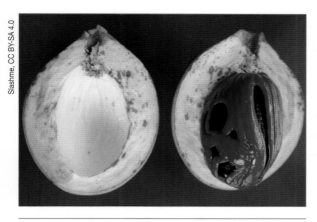

*Nutmeg seed (nut) and
red aril within the fruit*

merchants. Portugal had the monopoly of its trade until 1605, when the Dutch took over their possessions. The plantations were placed under military protection, and prices were kept high by systematic destruction of the trees growing on nearby islands. Huge amounts of the spice were even burned at intervals to keep the price high. Frenchman Pierre Poivre finally stole a few plants in 1768, and the nutmeg tree was then grown in other tropical countries.

Nutmeg has been highly appreciated since the early Middle Ages and was an ingredient of numerous balms, elixirs, and unguents. In 1704, Pollini wrote more than eight hundred pages on the invaluable virtues of nutmeg. He concluded that "in good health or disabled, alive or dead, nobody can do without this nut, the most salutary medicine!" It is indeed a very powerful tonic and stimulant.

Related organs: Digestive system

Medicinal properties: Tonic, stimulant (nervous system, circulation); digestive, intestinal antiseptic; sedative, analgesic; aphrodisiac; stupefying and toxic at high doses (delirium, hallucinations, fainting)

Indications: Digestive problems, intestinal infections, flatulence; asthenia; nervous and intellectual fatigue; impotence; rheumatic pain, neuralgia

MYRTACEAE
Harmony and Equilibrium in the Interaction of the Four Elements

Essential oils of this family include cajeput, clove, eucalyptus, myrtle, niaouli, and tea tree. Other oils of interest are allspice, bay, and red pepper. Myrtaceae grow in the tropical zones of every continent. Confronted with the powerful forces of earth and water in relation to strong tropical influences, Myrtaceae oppose a very structured formatting principle. The plants and trees of the family have a noble and harmonious aspect, which expresses the perfect equilibrium among the four elements (fire, air, water, earth) in the constitution of the type. The astral sphere is never violent to etheric formatting forces: the type does not produce any poisonous plant.

The family's evergreen leaves are strong and simple. They open themselves to the supra vegetal and animal sphere in an intense floral process (pollination is accomplished by insects and birds). The sugar process is very strong in this family, which produces some delicious fruits, such as pomegranate, gooseberry, guava, myrtle fruits, and jaboticaba plums.

The deep penetration of tropical warmth into the leaf, flower, bark, and wood generates etheric oils and aromatic resins. The family also

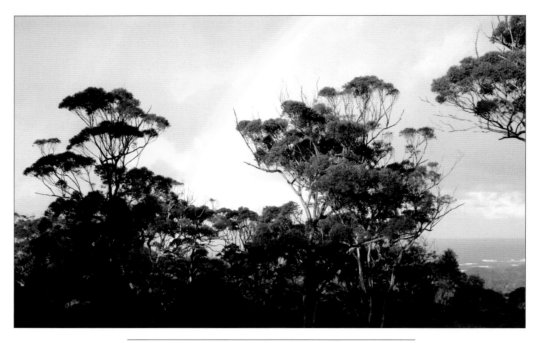

Eucalyptus

produces some condiments (cloves, red pepper). Finally, it produces very hard woods, which reveals the healthy relation of this family with the earth element.

Type of action: Re-equilibrating
Domain of action: Metabolism, energy centers, lungs
Indications: Respiratory diseases; metabolic or energetic lack of balance

Cajeput (*Melaleuca leucadendra*)

- Primarily produced in Malaysia and Far Eastern countries
- Essential oil is distilled from the leaves; it is yellowish green
- Fragrance: Penetrating and camphorlike
- Used in numerous pectoral preparations; also used as insecticide and parasiticide

In Malaysia and Java cajeput oil was a traditional remedy for cholera and rheumatism.

Medicinal properties: General antiseptic (pulmonary, urinary, intestinal); antispasmodic, antineuralgic; sudorific; febrifuge
Indications: Pulmonary diseases (bronchitis, tuberculosis); cystitis, urethritis; dysentery, diarrhea, amebiasis; rheumatism, rheumatic pains; earaches

Clove (*Eugenia caryophyllata*)

- Primarily produced in Molucca Islands, Madagascar, Zanzibar, and Indonesia

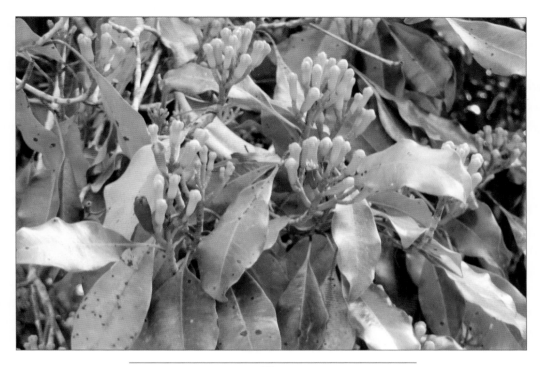

Clove

- Essential oil is distilled from the dried buds; it is brown to dark brown
- Essential oil is also distilled from clove stems and leaves but is of lower quality (especially oil from the stems); it is often used to adulterate clove bud oil
- Fragrance: Characteristically hot and spicy
- Used in dentistry, pharmacy, food industry, and perfumery

Native to the Molucca Islands, clove is one of the best-known spices of the world, along with black pepper, cinnamon, and nutmeg. It was so precious in ancient times that it caused a few wars: its trade was almost exclusively controlled by the Portuguese, who possessed the Molucca Islands until the seventeenth century, when the Dutch drove them out. To better control the monopoly and raise prices, the Dutch destroyed all plantations except the one on Ambon Island. The French finally stole a few plants to start new plantations in Guyana, Zanzibar, Réunion, and Trinidad. Clove oil was long used in dentistry as an analgesic.

In the clove tree, the terrestrial forces of the roots rise into the floral area: the essential oil of the buds, heavier than water and not easily volatile, is heavy and burning, which reveals that the fire cosmic forces have been strongly drawn into the ground. This special interaction of the fire and earth energies in the floral area results in a strong action on the metabolism: clove stimulates the digestion of heavy food and regulates the digestive tract.

Medicinal properties: Antineuralgic, analgesic; powerful antiseptic, cicatrizant; stomachic, carminative; aphrodisiac, stimulant; parasiticide

Indications: Toothache; prevention of infectious diseases; physical and intellectual asthenia (to strengthen memory); dyspepsia, gastric fermentation, flatulence; impotence; infected wounds, ulcers

Eucalyptus (*Eucalyptus globulus*)

- Primarily produced in Australia, Spain, and Portugal
- Essential oil is distilled from the leaves; it is yellow to red
- Fragrance: Fresh, balsamic, and camphor-like
- Numerous uses in pharmacy

Native to Australia, where it was regarded as a general cure-all by the Aborigines and later by the white settlers, eucalyptus has now spread almost entirely over the tropical and subtropical parts of the world. It has a long tradition of use in medicine, and its essential oil is one of the most powerful and versatile remedies. Eucalyptus is one of the tallest trees in the world and is deeply rooted: its roots go amazingly deep in the ground to find aquifer veins and strongly draw water to its vigorous branches and leaves. It is used to drain marshy areas and cleanse them from mosquitos. It grows incredibly fast but forms nevertheless a very strong wood that is fairly resistant to rot. The leaves, shaped like swords, are oriented in such a way as to avoid a strong exposure to the sun and allow the light to pass through the whole tree's growth and reach the ground. Eucalyptus energetically draws the solidifying forces of earth and water into the clear and dry area of air and light, where it attracts astral force for the production of essential oils—hence its action on the urinary and pulmonary systems. It is especially beneficent in the treatment of pulmonary inflammation and excessive mucosity.

Medicinal properties: General antiseptic (especially pulmonary and urinary); mucous fluidifier, expectorant, antispasmodic; hypoglycemic; febrifuge; stimulant; cicatrizant, vulnerary; parasiticide

Indications: Respiratory diseases (asthma, bronchitis, tuberculosis, flu, sinusitis); urinary infections; diabetes; fevers; rheumatism; intestinal parasites (ascarids, oxyurids)

Myrtle (*Myrtus communis*)

- Primarily produced in North Africa
- Essential oil is distilled from the branches; it is yellow

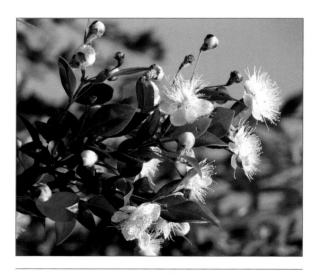

Myrtle

🌿 Fragrance: Fresh; close to eucalyptus

The Greeks and Romans used myrtle for pulmonary and urinary diseases. In the sixteenth century the leaves and flowers were used for skin care; they served in the preparation of "angel water," a renowned tonic and astringent lotion. The medicinal properties of myrtle closely resemble those of eucalyptus.

Specific therapeutic indications: Skin care

Niaouli (*Melaleuca viridiflora*)

🌿 Primarily produced in Madagascar, Australia, and New Caledonia

🌿 Essential oil (also called gomenol) is distilled from the leaves; it is yellow

🌿 Fragrance: Strong, camphorlike, and balsamic; close to eucalyptus

🌿 Same medicinal properties and indications as eucalyptus

Specific therapeutic indications: Stimulating to tissues (promotes local circulation and leukocyte and antibody activity); helpful for infected wounds, ulcers, and burns.

Tea Tree (*Melaleuca alternifolia*)

🌿 Primarily produced in Australia

🌿 Essential oil is distilled from the leaves; it is yellowish

🌿 Fragrance: Strong, camphorlike, balsamic, and pungent

Tea tree essential oil has become a universal panacea, first-aid kit, or cure-all. It is (with oregano and savory) one of the oils whose medical and antiseptic properties are the most widely documented. Research in Australia begun in the late 1920s showed the amazing anti-infectious power of the oil. During World War II it was even included in military first-aid kits in tropical areas. Extensive research during the 1970s and 1980s (by Morton Walker, Dr. Eduardo F. Pena, and Dr. Paul Belaiche, among others) showed its strong antifungal action. Its wide range of action and its low toxicity make it an ideal home remedy for inclusion in any aromatherapy first-aid kit (the same can be said of lavender and eucalyptus).

A somewhat small tree with needlelike leaves (similar to cypress), tea tree shows an amazing vitality. Before the demand for its oil increased dramatically beginning in the 1980s, tea tree was considered a weed—a real plague, in fact—and farmers could not get rid of it. Cut down to the roots, it regrows flourishing, thick foliage in less than two years. Even more than eucalyptus, it likes swampy, marshy areas. Unlike eucalyptus, though, its leaves are hardly developed, which indicates a predominance of earth, fire, and water over air. Tea tree yields one of the best antifungal, anti-infectious, and antiseptic oils, but eucalyptus works better on respiratory conditions. The amazing vitality of tea tree indicates its strong immunostimulant properties.

Medicinal properties: Antifungal (*Candida albicans, Trichomonas*); anti-infectious; general antiseptic (especially urinary); immunostimulant; mucus fluidifier, expectorant; cicatrizant, vulnerary; parasiticide

Indications: Fungal infections (ringworm, athlete's foot, vaginitis, thrush, *Candida albicans*);

urinary infections, cystitis; infected wounds, ulcers, sores, and any infectious condition; cold sores, blisters, chickenpox; acne; rashes, anal and genital pruritis, genital herpes; intestinal parasites; surgery preparation (prevention); low immune system; dandruff, hair care

OLEACEAE
Ethereal and Exquisite Creativity

Named after the fabled olive tree, the Oleaceae family of flowering shrubs, trees, and lianas includes some stunning ornamental plants with abundant, spectacular, and exquisitely fragrant blooming. Among these are examples of the most exquisite and refined fragrances of the vegetal realm, such as lilacs, jasmines, osmanthus, privet (*Ligustrum* spp.), and forsythia. Such fragrances are so delicate that they cannot withstand steam distillation and must be extracted by solvent or CO_2 extraction to produce absolutes.

In addition, members of the genus *Fraxinus* (ashes) are noted for their hardwood timber.

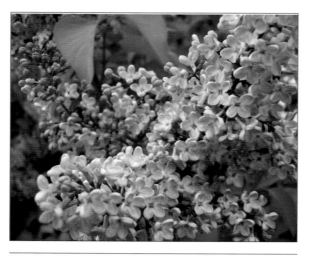

Lilac

Oleaceae are distributed throughout the world, except for the Arctic; they are especially abundant in tropical and temperate Asia. The tropical and warm-temperate species are evergreen; those from colder regions are deciduous.

Absolutes of this family include jasmine. Other absolutes of interest are osmanthus and lilac (CO_2 extraction).

Jasmine (*Jasminum officinalis*)

- Primarily produced in southern France, North Africa (Egypt, Tunisia, Morocco), and India
- There is no essential oil of jasmine; the absolute is obtained by either enfleurage or solvent extraction (see chapter 3), and it is brown and rather viscous
- Fragrance: Deep, sweet, warming, long-lasting, exhilarating, and supremely exotic
- Blends beautifully with rose, neroli, bergamot, petitgrain, sandalwood, citruses, palmarosa, geranium, and rosewood

With rose and neroli, jasmine is one of the major "noble" oils of perfumery. It is also one of the most expensive oils; therefore it is very often adulterated. If rose is the oil of love, jasmine is certainly the oil of romance and was revered as such in the Hindu and Muslim traditions. It inspired burning lascivious songs by the Arab poets. In the harem, the prince's favorite soaked in a jasmine-scented bath and received an elaborate jasmine massage to induce sensual ecstasy in her lover.

Supremely sensual, jasmine is certainly the best aphrodisiac that aromatherapy can offer. It should not be considered a mere sexual stim-

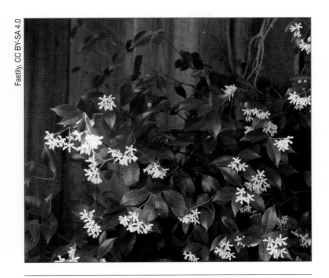

Jasmine

ulant, though. Jasmine releases inhibition, liberates imagination, and develops exhilarating playfulness. In a way the power of jasmine can only be fully experienced by real lovers, as it has the power to transcend physical love and fully release sexual energy. It is the best stimulant of the sacral (sexual) chakra and is recommended for any type of kundalini work.

Medicinal properties: Aphrodisiac, stimulant of sacral chakra; antidepressant; childbirth preparation
Indications: Impotence, frigidity; anxiety, depression, lethargy, lack of confidence; postnatal depression; makes a fine perfume

PIPERACEAE
The Pepper Family

The Piperaceae, or pepper, family are a large family of flowering herbs, vines, shrubs, and trees widely distributed throughout the tropics and subtropics, with two main genera: *Piper* (2,000 species) and *Peperomia* (1,600 species). Their leaves and fruits have a pungent flavor that can be attributed to their constituents chavicine, piperine, and piperidine. Fruits are drupe-like, with a single seed per fruit.

Native to southern India and Sri Lanka, *Piper nigrum* is a tall woody climber that yields most of the peppercorns that are used as spices, including black and white pepper.

Many Piperaceae are used in medicines and in food and beverages as spices and seasonings. Cubeb (*Piper cubeba*), grown in Southeast Asia for its fruit and essential oil, is used in various medicines and for flavoring cigarettes and bitters. Betel pepper (*Piper betle*) is chewed with slices of betel nut (*Areca catechu*) and lime as a mild stimulant. Pacific Islanders prepare a ceremonial drink known as *kava* or *kawakawa* from the root of *Piper methysticum,* which has narcotic and sedative effects.

Pepper (*Piper nigrum*)
- Primarily produced in India, Java, Sumatra, and China
- Essential oil is distilled from the seeds; it is yellow green
- Fragrance: Characteristic
- Few uses in perfumery or food industry

One of the most ancient spices, pepper was mentioned in Chinese and Sanskrit texts a few thousand years ago. In the Western countries it was the most valued spice and was used as currency in the Middle Ages. The essential oil of pepper was described by Valerius Cordius

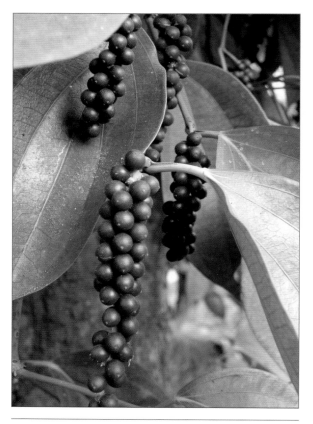

Pepper

in his *Compendium Aromatorium* in 1488. It is traditionally indicated as a stimulant and tonic and whenever there is an excess of cold or water.

Medicinal properties: Stimulant, tonic (especially for the digestive and nervous systems); digestive, stomachic, antitoxic; heating, drying, comforting; analgesic, rubefacient; aphrodisiac; stimulant of the root chakra

Indications: Digestive problems (dyspepsia, flatulence, loss of appetite, food poisoning); fever, cold, catarrh, cough, influenza; neuralgia, toothache, rheumatic aches; muscular pain, sport

massage (in preparation for competition); gonorrhea; impotence; ungroundedness

POACEAE (GRAMINAE)
The Nutritious Family

Essential oils of this family include citronella, lemongrass, palmarosa, and vetiver. A wide majority of the plants covering the ground belong to the Poaceae family. From the poles to the equator, from the swamps to the deserts, this family shows an amazing adaptability and diversity. Its ability to cover almost exclusively huge areas denotes a singular strength. This strength lies in its powerful root system, which forms an intricate network that blends almost perfectly with the soil (to create lawns, modern gardeners lay on the soil a kind of carpet that is vegetal and ground together). Above this intense root system, the aerial part of Poaceae is dominated by a linear principle: long narrow leaves and straight stems. Even the inflorescence (ear) obeys this principle.

This family does not spend much energy in the floral process. It is entirely dedicated to another aim: nutrition. Its leaves and seeds are a gift to the animal kingdom, with grass for herbivores and grain (wheat, rice, corn, barley, oats) for rodents, birds, and humans.

Poaceae has the potential to develop fragrances—like the scent of freshly cut hay! But it usually remains a potential, nascent fragrance. Only under the tropics has this ability been fully developed in some species. The herbs of citronella, lemongrass, and palmarosa have a fresh, green, lemony, slightly rosy fra-

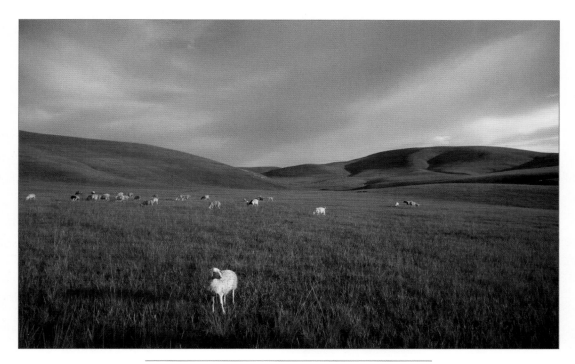

Poaceae prairie—gift to the animal kingdom

grance. Vetiver produces essential oils in its roots.

Citronella (*Cymbopogon nardus*)

🍃 Primarily produced in China, Malaysia, Sri Lanka, and Central America

🍃 Essential oil is distilled from the herb; it is yellow

🍃 Fragrance: Fresh, green, and lemony

🍃 Widely used in the soap industry, deodorizers, insecticide, and sanitary products; few uses in perfumery

Medicinal properties and indications: Disinfection of rooms; insecticide

Lemongrass (*Cymbopogon citratus*)

🍃 Primarily produced in India, Central America, and Brazil

🍃 Essential oil is distilled from the herb; it is yellow to reddish brown

🍃 Fragrance: Fresh and lemony; finer than citronella

🍃 Widely used in the soap industry and in perfumery; a traditional culinary herb in China

According to the Indian pharmacopoeia, lemongrass was traditionally used as an antidote against infectious diseases, fevers, and cholera.

Medicinal properties: Stimulant of the digestive system (stomachic, carminative, digestive); antiseptic; diuretic; insect repellent

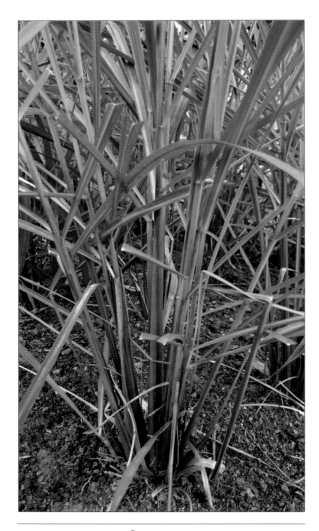

Lemongrass

Indications: Digestive troubles (dyspepsia, colic, flatulence); disinfection, deodorization; pediculosis, scabies

Veterinary uses: Parasites, digestive troubles

Palmarosa (*Cymbopogon martinii*)

- Primarily produced in India, Africa, Comoro Islands, and Madagascar

- Essential oil is distilled from the herb; it is yellow
- Fragrance: Fresh and roselike
- Widely used in perfumery and cosmetology (and to adulterate or dilute rose essential oil, one of the most expensive essential oils)

Medicinal properties: Antiseptic; cellular stimulant; hydrating; febrifuge; digestive stimulant

Indications: Skin care—wrinkles, acne, and the like (reestablishes the physiological balance of the skin, immediate calming and refreshing action); digestive atonia

Vetiver (*Andropogon muricatus*)

- Primarily produced in Comoro Islands, Caribbean Islands, and Réunion
- Essential oil is distilled from the roots; it is deep brown and very thick
- Fragrance: Deep, hearty, woody (slightly reminiscent of tobacco plant or clary sage), musky, and sandalwood-like
- Used mostly in perfumery and cosmetics; makes a very good fixative

With vetiver, the aromatic process is drawn into the roots, wherein lies the power of Poaceae. Its fragrance is then an actualization in the odoriferous sphere of the potentialities that the type usually expresses in the nutritious sphere. The characteristic earthy, realistic, almost materialistic scent definitively accounts for the nutritious aspect of the family, while the musky note reminds one of its animal connection.

Poaceae produce the most sacred food of the vegetable kingdom: wheat, rice, and corn—

food beyond food, gift of the gods to the human realm. Vetiver expresses this fundamental aspect of the type through its sandalwood-like note; it is inspiring and uplifting.

Indication: Arthritis

ROSACEAE
The Quest for Perfection

With more than 4,800 known species of herbs, shrubs, and trees in ninety genera distributed worldwide, the rose family (Rosaceae) is the third most economically important angiosperm family, after the Poaceae (grasses and grains) and Fabaceae (legumes, peas, beans, alfalfa, etc). Usually divided into three subfamilies (Amygdaloideae, Dryadoideae, and Rosoideae), it produces a vast array of delicious fruits: strawberry, raspberry, blackberry, boysenberry, almond, plum, peach, apricot, nectarine, cherry, blackthorn, apple, crab apple, pear, quince, hawthorn, loquat, rose hip, and so on, with all their subspecies and varieties.

The Rosaceae also include many important ornamental trees and shrubs, such as roses, of course, as well as cherry trees (of cherry-blossom fame), meadowsweets, photinias, firethorns, rowans, and hawthorns.

All Rosaceae of commercial value, whether fruits or ornamentals, have evolved dramatically from their wild relatives, increasing in size, sweetness, appearance, or other desirable attributes as a result of their interactive coevolution with the humans. Domestication led to constant selection, hybridization, grafting, cloning, and other propagation techniques, resulting in

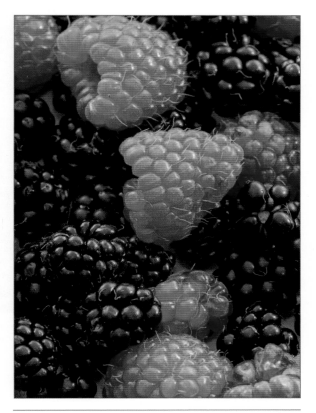

Raspberries and blackberries of the Rosaceae family

accelerated evolution that created the commercial Rosaceae with which we are familiar.

To the best of my knowledge, rose is the only plant among the Roasaceae from which essential oil is produced, but with rose, the family comes as close to perfection as any plant can be in the botanical realm. Its flower is almost universally revered as a symbol of pure love, mysticism, and devotion. Rose is a symbol of the Virgin Mary and is often associated with sainthood and angels in Christianity. Its fragrance is one of the most highly prized by perfumers and aromatherapists alike.

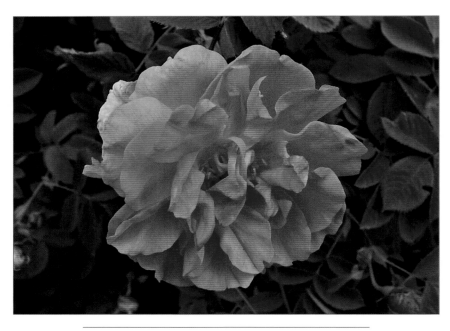

Rosa damascena

Rose (*Rosa centifolia and R. damascena*)

🌿 Primarily produced in Bulgaria, Morocco, and Turkey

🌿 Rosebuds are picked during a few morning hours only, right after the dew, and distilled immediately; the essential oil is rather thick and yellow to greenish yellow

🌿 Fragrance: Characteristic

One of the most expensive essential oils, rose oil is almost always adulterated with substances like geranium, lemongrass, palmarosa, and terpene alcohols (geraniol, citronellol, rhodinol, linalool, nerol, etc.). The processes of adulteration have become so refined that is almost impossible to disclose frauds. Real rose oil is used only in very high-grade perfumes. Rose water is widely used in cosmetics and perfumery.

Whether it sprang from the blood of Venus, the blood of Adonis, or the sweat of Mohammed, the rose—the queen of flowers—is certainly immemorial. Praised by the poets, revered in the sacred books, and offered to the kings and the gods, the rose is a traditional symbol of love. Bunches of roses were found in the sarcophagus of Tutankhamun, offered by Queen Ankhsenamon as a token of her love. When the Persian emperor Djihanguyr married the princess Nour-Djihan, a canal encircling the gardens was filled with rose water. Droplets of oil were noticed floating on the top of the water—that is said to have been the beginning of the production of the famous Persian rose oil.

Rose water is an excellent skin tonic, recommended for any type of skin; it is good for wrinkles, inflammation, redness, and sensitive skin and is indicated for ophthalmia.

Related organs: Female reproductive system
Medicinal properties: Uplifting, antidepressant, tonic; astringent, hemostatic; depurative; aphrodisiac; stimulant of the heart chakra
Indications: Nervous tension, depression, insomnia, headache; skin care (wrinkles, eczema, sensitive skin, aged skin); disorders of the female reproductive system (frigidity, sterility, uterine disorders); hemorrhage; impotence; emotional shock, grief, depression

RUTACEAE
Processes of Subdued Topical Heat

Essential oils of this family include bergamot, grapefruit, lemon, lime, neroli, orange, petitgrain, and tangerine. Other oils of interest are rue (*Ruta graveolens*)—though note that rue essential oil is highly toxic and should be used only with great care.

Most Rutaceae grow in tropical areas; here, they are mostly small thorny trees with hard wood, which is often resinous, and firm green leaves. Their beautiful abundant flowers are shaped like symmetrical stars and exhale a delicious, sweet, slightly exhilarating fragrance. The scent of the leaves is fresh and comforting, with a hint of bitterness. The trees develop juicy acid fruits (citrus) or small, hot, spicy berries.

The general therapeutic activity of Rutaceae concerns the interaction of warmth and fluid in the body. The oils reduce proliferations, distensions, inflammations, and looseness; they strengthen the astral body, and their formatting

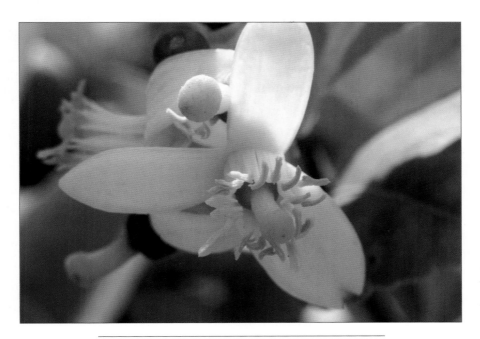

Rutaceae, citrus blossom

forces are activated by air and warmth.

Many members of the genus *Citrus* are listed and discussed here. Distillation of the flowers of bitter orange yields neroli essential oil; cistillation of the leaves gives petitgrain. The essential oils of bergamot, grapefruit, lemon, lime, orange, and tangerine are extracted from the peel of the fruits by cold pressure.

Extremely prolific (each tree can produce up to a hundred fruits), deeply rooted, and densely ramified, citruses perfectly control the interaction of the two powerful opposite flows of forces: centrifugal forces that strongly draw up the terrestrial forces, charging them with vitalized fluid elements of a tropical luxuriance, and cosmic forces of light and warmth that are absorbed by the leaves, the bark, the wood, and the fruit. Their energetic floral process and their light, suave, almost ethereal and very pervasive fragrance suggest an etheric organism intensely penetrated by the peripheral astral sphere. Citrus fruits are liquid, like a berry, but are surrounded with a tough envelope shaped by the forces of air and warmth.

Citruses strive against the dissolving centrifugal forces of the tropical world. Their action is refreshing, vivifying, and tonic and tends to gather the constitutive elements of the body.

The floral area expresses a soft, delicious, appeasing exhilaration, indicative of the remarkable sedative, antidepressant power of the blossoms. The fragrance of the thick, vigorous leaves is less refined, more hearty and grounded, and slightly bitter. The leaves' action is then invig-

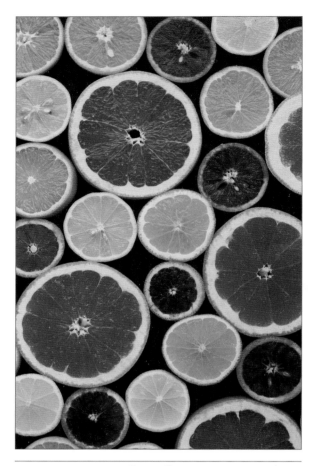

Citrus fruits

orating, comforting, and almost materialistic, even compared with the ethereal neroli.

Type of action: Cooling, refreshing; sedative (flowers); control of liquid processes and secretion (fruits)

Domain of action: Digestive system, kidneys, liver; nervous system

Indications: Inflammations, infectious diseases; excess of liquids (obesity); oversensitivity, nervous tension

Bergamot (*Citrus bergamia*)

- Primarily produced in Italy, the Ivory Coast, and Guinea
- Essential oil is extracted by cold pressure of the rind of the fruit; it is yellowish green to emerald
- Fragrance: Sweet and citrusy, with a floral note
- Widely used in perfumery; blends perfectly with almost any oil; makes a perfect top note

Medicinal properties: Antispasmodic; antiseptic; cordial, tonic, stomachic, digestive; vulnerary

Indications: Colic, intestinal infection, intestinal parasites, stomatitis; skin care

Grapefruit (*Citrus paradisi*)

- Primarily produced in the United States
- Essential oil is extracted by cold pressure of the rind of the fruit; it is yellow
- Various uses in perfumery and food industry
- Blends fairly well with other citrus oils, geranium, and cedarwood

Specific therapeutic indications: Obesity

Lemon (*Citrus limon*)

- Produced all around the Mediterranean and in California, Brazil, and Argentina
- Essential oil is extracted by cold pressure of the rind of the fruit; it is yellow to yellowish green
- Numerous uses in perfumery, cosmetics, pharmacy, and the food and soap industries
- Blends well with many oils; makes a nice green note
- One of the most versatile essential oils in aromatherapy

Profusely thorny, with very thick leaves and the most acid fruit of the vegetable kingdom, the small lemon tree gives an impression of fresh, optimistic, fearless strength. Here the fire/water dialectic is resolved on the cooling side. The fruit is tightly structured under a fairly tough skin; expansion, dilation, and inflation are under control.

Medicinal properties: Bactericidal, antiseptic, stimulant of leukocytosis; stimulant, tonic; stomachic, carminative; diuretic; hepatic; liquefies the blood, hypotensive agent; depurative; antirheumatic

Indications: Infectious diseases; anemia, asthenia; varicosis, arteriosclerosis, hyperviscosity of the blood, hypertension; rheumatism; dyspepsia, flatulence; hepatic congestion; skin diseases, skin care; herpes

Lime (*Citrus aurantifolia*)

- Primarily produced in Florida, Central America, and Caribbean Islands
- Essential oil is extracted from the rind of the fruit by cold pressure or distillation. The cold-pressed oil is far superior to the distilled oil; it is gold to yellowish green
- Fragrance: Fresh, green, and very pleasant; similar to bergamot for the cold-pressed oil; much heavier for the distilled oil

The indications and various uses of lime are similar to those of lemon (although its refreshing quality is more pronounced). It makes a very good aftershave lotion.

Neroli (*Citrus aurantium*)

- Primarily produced in France, Spain, North Africa, Italy, and the Comoro Islands
- Essential oil is distilled from the blossoms of the bitter orange tree and has a golden color
- One of the most expensive oils, and therefore widely adulterated
- Fragrance: One of the finest floral essences; sweet, suave, delicious, and slightly euphoric
- Used in expensive cologne and perfumes; blends well with almost any oil and is useful as the heart of a floral blend

Real neroli (also called neroli biguarade) is extracted from the blossom of bitter orange (biguarade). However, blossoms of other citruses (sweet orange, lemon, mandarin) are also sometimes distilled. Native to China, where its flowers were traditionally used in cosmetics, bitter orange now grows all around the Mediterranean, in the United States, and in Central and South America. Neroli essential oil was already being produced by the beginning of the sixteenth century. It became a fashionable perfume when the Duchess of Nerole started using it to scent her gloves.

The hydrolate obtained by distillation of bitter orange blossom is more commonly known as orange-flower water; it is widely used for skin care and pastry making. It is soothing, digestive, and carminative.

Medicinal properties: Antidepressant, antispasmodic, sedative; diminishes the amplitude of heart muscle contractions; aphrodisiac; stimulant of the heart chakra

Indications: Insomnia, hysteria, anxiety, depression, nervous tension; palpitations; diarrhea related to stress; skin care (dry or sensitive skin); grief, emotional shock; mild remedy for infants' colic and to send them to sleep

Sweet Orange (*Citrus aurantium*)

- Primarily produced in Spain, North Africa, the United States, and Central and South America
- Essential oil is extracted by cold pressure of the rind of the fruit; it is orange
- Numerous uses in perfumery and food industry

Biguarade, or bitter orange, is even more thorny than lemon; the strong bitterness of its fruit indicates a special affinity for the liver. With sweet orange, qualities are softened: no more thorns, and the fruit is now totally edible. The water processes are less tight, and the soothing properties are more pronounced.

Medicinal properties: Febrifuge; stomachic, digestive; antispasmodic, sedative, cardiotonic
Indications: Fever; indigestion, dyspepsia, flatulence, gastric spasms; skin care, wrinkles, dermatitis; nervous troubles

Petitgrain (*Citrus aurantium*)

- Primarily produced in France, Spain, North Africa, Italy, and the Comoro Islands
- Essential oil is distilled from the leaves of the bitter orange tree; it is slightly golden
- Fragrance: Fresh, invigorating, and slightly floral, with a bitter note

- Widely used in pharmacy and perfumery (the basic ingredient of good colognes); blends well with almost any oil

Real petitgrain (or petitgrain biguarade) is obtained by distilling the leaves of the bitter orange (biguarade) tree. Petitgrain bergamot, petitgrain lemon, and petitgrain mandarin are also produced.

Specific therapeutic indications: Painful digestion; sedative of nervous system; tonic, intellectual stimulant, strengthens memory

Mandarin and Tangerine (*Citrus reticulata*)

- Primarily produced in Italy (mandarin) and the United States (tangerine)
- Essential oil is extracted by cold pressure of the rind of the fruit; it is dark orange
- The essential oil of mandarin is much finer than that of tangerine (a hybrid)
- Fragrance: Sweeter than orange; reminiscent of bergamot

Native to China, mandarin is the most delicate fruit; it was traditionally offered to the mandarins (hence its name). Its medicinal properties are very close to those of orange. The sedative and antispasmodic properties, however, are more pronounced.

Mandarin is certainly the softest of all citrus trees. The leaves are delicate, the fruit is very sweet, and the taste is quite refined. The peel is soft and the fragrance is almost exotic. The soothing action on the nervous centers is then quite pronounced. The same can be said for tangerine, which is a type of mandarin.

Specific therapeutic indications: Calming, antispasmodic; alleviates nervous tension, insomnia, epilepsy

SANTALACEAE

The Spiritual Family

Santalaceae, the sandalwood family, counts about thirty-six genera and more than four hundred species of semiparasitic flowering herbs, shrubs, climbers, and trees that are widely distributed in tropical and temperate regions. Though their green leaves contain some chlorophyll, allowing the plants to photosynthesize some of their own nutrients, all Santalaceae are parasites to a certain extent and rely on their hosts for water and nutrients. Most, including sandalwood, are root parasites; the others are stem parasites.

Most Santalaceae have tiny bisexual or unisexual flowers and bear one-seeded fruits often surrounded by a brightly colored nutlike structure. Some of the fruits are edible, most notably quandong (*Santalum acuminatum*).

Indian sandalwood (*Santalum album*) and its close relatives, the Australian sandalwood (*Santalum spicatum*) and New Caledonian sandalwood (*Santalum austrocaledonicum*), are the only Santalaceae of commercial value. All have become endangered in the wild due to overharvesting.

Red sandalwood (*Pterocarpus santalinus*), though it bears the sandalwood name, belongs to the Fabaceae family and is not botanically related.

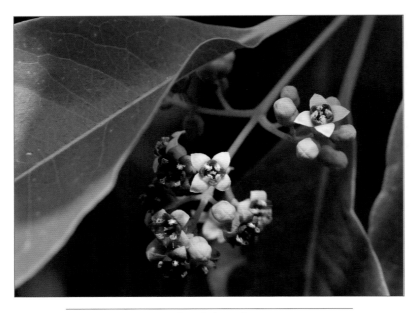

Sandalwood

The Viscaceae (mistletoes) are sometimes considered a subfamily of the Santalaceae.

Sandalwood (*Santalum album*)

- Primarily produced in India, Indonesia, and China
- Essential oil is distilled from the inner wood; it is thick and yellow
- Fragrance: Characteristic (persistent, woody, sweet, and spicy)
- Very good fixative, widely used in high-class perfumes; often adulterated

A sacred tree of India, sandalwood is mentioned in ancient Sanskrit and Chinese texts. It is widely used as incense, in religious ceremonies, and in medicine and cosmetics. The Mysore district of Karnataka in India produces the most valued sandalwood in the world. Mysore sandalwood has become endangered in recent years and its export is strictly controlled.

Sandalwood is one of the greatest essential oils for blending, acting as a base note and fixative and imparting a deep, woody, exotic, smooth tone to any blend. Considering its endangered status, its scarcity, and its price, its use should be restrained to emotional, mental, and spiritual applications.

Sandalwood promotes alertness and is anxiolytic and relaxant. It can reach deep into the soul and help soothe emotional wounds and open up spiritual channels.

Indian sandalwood (*Santalum album*) was traditionally used for furniture, incense, and perfumery. It is now rare and endangered in the wild, having been overharvested in most of India's forests. Scarcity has led to a price explosion exacerbated by poor enforcement of arcane regulations and corruption, leading itself to widespread smuggling, in a vicious circle to near extinction.

Cultivation is challenging as germination is unpredictable and the plant, being semiparasitic, must anchor on the root system of host trees. The best quality and highest yields require forty-year-old trees in the wild, with the very finest coming from eighty-year-old trees. The cycle can be reduced to fifteen years in cultivation.

Santalum spicatum, the Australian sandalwood, a tree native to semiarid areas at the edge of southwest Australia, is a potential candidate for substitution for *S. album.* It has been severely depleted in the wild due to overharvesting and deforestation, but large-scale cultivation was successfully launched at the turn of the millennium, with more than 10,000 hectares in cultivation as of 2019, and rapid expansion. The first harvest came in 2014.

Related organs: Genitourinary tract

Medicinal properties: Genitourinary antiseptic, diuretic; antidepressant, tonic, aphrodisiac; antispasmodic; astringent

Indications: Genitourinary infections (gonorrhea, blennorrhoea, cystitis, colibacillosis); impotence

VERBENACEAE
The Vervain Family

The Verbenaceae, the verbena or vervain family, is a family of mainly tropical flowering plants with thirty genera and some 1,100 species, some of which are cultivated as ornamentals. They have opposite or whorled leaves, usually undivided. Their flowers, many of which are aromatic, are aggregated in spikes, clusters, or racemes.

The shrub lemon verbena (*Aloysia triphylla*) is widely used as herbal tea and notable for

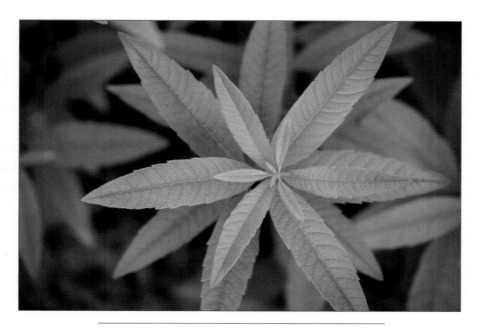

Lemon verbena

its essential oil. The family also includes teak (*Tectona grandis*), native to Southeast Asia, which is one of the most valuable timber trees in the world.

Lemon Verbena (*Lippia citriodora* or *Aloysia triphylla*)

🌿 Primarily produced in southern France and North Africa

🌿 Essential oil is distilled from the leaves and branches; it is yellowish green

🌿 Fragrance: Fresh and lemony; similar to lemongrass but more refined

There is much confusion about verbena oil; many essential oils are improperly called verbena. Indian verbena, for example, is actually a variety of lemongrass (from the Poaceae family), while exotic verbena is *Litsea cubeba* (from the Lauraceae family).

Native to Chile and Peru, true lemon verbena is a small bush with an abundant leaf system. The leaves and branches are steam distilled for the production of the oil. The yield is very low, making true lemon verbena essential oil rather rare and expensive. The world production of the *essential* oil is limited and represents only a fraction of the total sales of the oil (you can guess where the rest comes from). Lemon verbena is a lovely oil that gives a nice fresh lemony top note to blends. It is best used in a diffuser.

Medicinal properties: Liver and digestive stimulant; cooling, refreshing, febrifuge; antidepressant; calming at low doses

Indications: Nervousness, insomnia, tachycardia; digestive troubles

ZINGIBERACEAE
The Spicy Family

Zingiberaceae, the ginger family, has about fifty-two genera and more than 1,300 species distributed in moist areas of the tropics and subtropics. These flowering aromatic perennial herbaceous plants have creeping horizontal or tuberous rhizomes and grow up to 6 meters. The overlapping rolled-up sheathing at the base of the leaves sometimes forms a short pseudo aerial stem. The family includes some important ornamental plants producing spectacular flowers with bright colors and unusual shapes.

The Zingiberaceae include a large number of medicinal plants and play a major role in Ayurvedic medicine, the traditional medicine of India. They produce some of the most important spices of Asian cuisine, like ginger, cardamom, galangal, and turmeric. They are an important source of essential oils and oleoresins for aromatherapy, perfumery, and the food industry.

Essential oils of this family include ginger. Other oils of interest are cardamom, galangal, and turmeric.

Ginger (*Zingiber officinale*)

🌿 Primarily produced in China, India, and Malaysia

🌿 Essential oil is distilled from the rhizome; it is slightly yellow to dark yellow

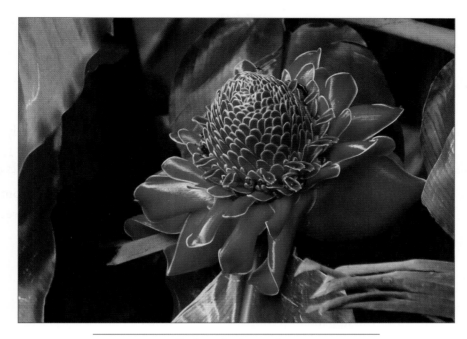

Red torch ginger plant

- Fragrance: Characteristic (camphor-like, aromatic, and citrusy)
- Widely used in the East (especially India, China, Japan) in pharmaceutical preparations; many uses in the food and beverage industries

Ginger has been used for thousands of years in India and China for its remarkable medicinal properties and for its culinary benefits. It is still one of the major remedies prescribed by macrobiotic therapists and Chinese doctors. Dioscorides recommended it for digestion and stomach weakness. It was mentioned in the Middle Ages as a tonic, stimulant, and febrifuge. It is also an ingredient of the balm of Fioraventi.

Related organs: Digestive system
Medicinal properties: Tonic, stimulant; stomachic, carminative; analgesic; febrifuge; antiscorbutic

Indications: Deficiency of the digestive system (dyspepsia, flatulence, loss of appetite, etc.); impotence; rheumatic pain

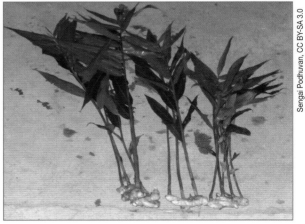

Ginger plants with rhizomes

TEN

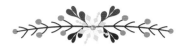

Aromatic Choreography

The Art and Science of Aromatic Composition

All essential oils and aromatherapy products act on several levels, from the biochemical and physical effects to the subtlest psychological, emotional, energetic, and spiritual effects. To maximize the aromatherapeutic power, all of these effects must act in synergy. This is especially the case for skin care products, especially those intended for facial care, the nose being at the center of the face.

True beauty is a perception, an attitude, a way of being, and the way a beauty product makes you feel is a fundamental part of its effects. It is inconceivable for a beauty product to have an unpleasant odor; if it did, it would not *be* a beauty product.

THE ART OF BLENDING

In this chapter we will explore the art of aromatic choreography—that is, combining essential oils to create a blend in which all the parts come together, therapeutically and aesthetically, in an aromatic composition akin to an olfactory ballet or a fragrance orchestration.

Consider Maurice Ravel's *Boléro,* one of the most famous musical works in the classical repertoire. It is based on a simple rhythm, which is repeated throughout the work, and two melodies, also very simple, that repeat themselves crescendo eight times before the final climax. The bolero is a useful metaphor for the art of aromatic composition in several aspects. First, it shows us that a masterpiece does not have to be complicated; on the contrary, it can be exceedingly simple. Second, the structure of the work is interesting, as it is built in layers, arising from a very simple theme, with each layer based on the previous one. It should be noted that Ravel did not consider *Boléro* to be real music; to him, it was just an experiment, "an orchestral fabric without music."

Master perfumers may blend more than a hundred aromatic compounds to create a perfume, but following the musical metaphor of the *Boléro,* simplicity is often preferable for

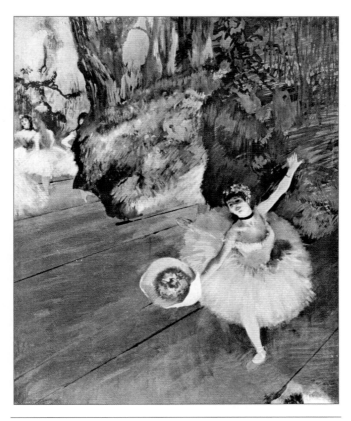

Dancer with a Bouquet of Flowers *by Edgar Degas, 1878*

blending purposes, especially for beginners.

As we have seen, aromatherapy acts on different levels (see fig. 6.1, page 58):

✦ On the physical level, essential oils can cure many common diseases. They are formed of very small molecules that are readily absorbed through the skin and penetrate the body. They act physiologically as antiseptics, antispasmodics, and analgesics, among other properties; they can stimulate organs and systems, such as the liver, the respiratory system, and so on.

✦ Essential oils have a profound action on the energetic level.

✦ Essential oils deeply affect our emotions and the psyche through their interaction with the olfactory system. The olfactory system is the most primitive part of the brain and is closely linked to memory and emotions.

✦ On the spiritual level, essential oils can have a profound effect in lifting our minds to higher planes. Sandalwood, benzoin, cistus, incense, and myrrh have been used since time immemorial to facitlitate spiritual rituals, ceremonies, and meditation.

More importantly, aromatherapy has a definitive ludic, Dionysiac dimension to it—it is playful, joyful, lightening, and heartening. Unlike allopathic medicine, where you often must suffer first to deserve your recovery, enjoyment is part of the aromatic treatment!

Blending is the most creative part of aromatherapy; it is an art. Like any art, it requires a balance of practice and intuition. There are some basic rules, but rules will not create a masterpiece without the proper dose of intuition. Blending is also what makes aromatherapy such a powerful therapeutic tool. You can blend essential oils targeted to treat specific needs or issues, enhancing the effectiveness of your treatments.

For the amateur as well as the professional, blending is one of most enjoyable aspects of aromatherapy. It can, in fact, become a very enjoyable hobby. Just like you don't have to be a virtuoso to enjoy violin or piano, you don't have to be a master perfumer to enjoy blending. You might occasionally offend the nose of some of your friends, especially in the beginning, but you'll also have fun and learn from your mistakes.

Nature has created hundreds of essential oils. In practice you can readily find on the marketplace fifty to eighty of the most common oils (such as lavender, eucalyptus, lemon, bergamot, cedarwood, and ylang-ylang) and some more exotic and unusual ones (such as cistus, everlasting, lovage, and melissa). While there are a number of reputable sources offering a wide variety of essential oils, you can use the art of blending to have access to infinite variations.

THE CONCEPT OF SYNERGY

Just like almost anything that deals with life forces, aromatherapy does not abide by the laws of arithmetic. The whole is not the sum of its parts. Two plus two does not necessarily equal four; it might equal three or five, or sometimes even ten! The situation in which the whole is greater than the sum of its parts is called a synergy.

Some essential oils have mutually enhancing powers, while others inhibit each other. A combination of mutually enhancing oils is called a synergy. Synergies help the therapist to be very accurate and precise in the treatment.

Creating synergies is the most important part of blending, requiring a deep understanding of essential oils, a fair amount of experience, and a lot of intuition. Intuition and experience are very important because synergies are rather context dependent. A given combination of oils might be an excellent synergy for one patient, but totally inappropriate for another.

To create a good synergy, you need to take into account not only the symptoms that you want to treat, but also the underlying causes of the disorder, the biological terrain, and the psychological or emotional factors involved.

All this may sound discouraging to the beginner, but if you follow some basic rules, you will be able to create decent blends.

1. Do not blend more than three or four oils at a time in the beginning; wait until you've gained some experience.

2. Do not blend oils with opposite effects (like a calming and a stimulant). Check thoroughly the properties of the oils that you want to blend and make sure that they complement each other for the particular patient you are treating.

3. A blend has to be pleasant to your patient. This is possibly the most important part of blending. Once you have selected the oils that will be efficient in treating your patient's condition, look at their fragrance compatibility and adjust your blend accordingly.

Below I have given some basic rules about proportions. I have also provided some basic blends that can be used advantageously for common ailments.

THE PRINCIPLES OF BLENDING

For blending purposes, essential oils are classified into top notes, middle notes, and base notes. A good fragrance composition should harmoniously balance these three categories. When I blend, I use an additional set of classifications: equalizers, modifiers, and enhancers, as well as fixatives.

Fragrance classification is bound to be highly subjective. Different authors might disagree on the classification of certain oils. Although, for most of my presentation, I systematically checked my information against other people's findings, I generally relied upon my own knowledge and experience of the oils to establish the classifications. I encourage you to develop your own categories and classifications as you become more experienced with essential oils and blending. Systems of classification are tools and should be used as such. If you find a system that works better for you, do not hesitate to use it.

Top Notes

Top notes will hit you first in a fragrance. They do not last very long, but they are very important in a blend, because they give the first impression of the blend. Top notes are sharp, penetrating, volatile, extreme, and either cold or hot, but never warm. From a chemical point of view, they are found mostly in the aldehydes and the esters. In the plant they are found in flowers, leaves, and fruits.

Typical top notes include bergamot, petitgrain, neroli, lemon, lime, orange (all citruses, in fact), lemongrass, peppermint, thyme, cinnamon, and clove (see table 17 on page 155). While certain top notes can be used rather liberally (lemon, bergamot, petitgrain), the sharpest ones (cinnamon, cloves, thyme) should be used in very small amounts. Top notes should constitute 20 to 40 percent of your blend. Diffuser blends can use larger amounts of top notes.

Middle Notes

Middle notes give body to your blends; they smooth the sharp edges and round the corners. They are warm, round, soft, and mellow. They are often "blend enhancers"—that is, oils to add to your blend less for their medicinal properties than for their fragrant qualities (for more on blend enhancers, keep reading). Monoterpene alcohols are typically middle notes. They are mostly found in leaves and herbs.

Typical middle notes are rosewood, geranium, lavender, chamomile, and marjoram (see table 17). Middle notes usually form the bulk of a blend (40 to 80 percent).

Base Notes

Base notes deepen your blend and increase its lasting effect. Base notes are warm, rich, and mostly pleasant. Most of them have traditional ritual uses. They generally affect the chakras and have deep effects on the mental, emotional, and spiritual planes and on the astral body. When smelled from the bottle, base notes may seem rather faint, but, when applied to the skin, they react strongly and release their power, which lasts for several hours.

Typical base notes are sandalwood, clary sage, frankincense, vanilla, benzoin, cedarwood, and spruce (see table 17). They are found mostly in woods and gums and are typically sesquiterpenes.

While base notes are not really necessary for a diffuser blend (although they do add depth to it), they are almost mandatory in any preparation to be applied to the skin. They can be used as 10 to 25 percent of a blend.

Fixatives

Even deeper than base notes and often grouped with them, fixatives draw your blend into the skin, giving it roots and permanence. They are necessary for long-lasting effect and are deep, intense, and profound. Some animal fixatives,

such as musk or civet, can last for days. Typical fixatives are cistus, myrrh, patchouli, and vetiver (see table 17).

The first hit of a fixative is not necessarily very pleasant (musk and civet are definitively obnoxious, while patchouli is unpleasant to many people and vetiver and cistus may seem weird), but no decent perfume could be made without them. Fixatives should be used sparingly to avoid overpowering the blend (they rarely account for more than 5 percent of any blend). They are found in roots and gums and are sesquiterpenes or diterpenes.

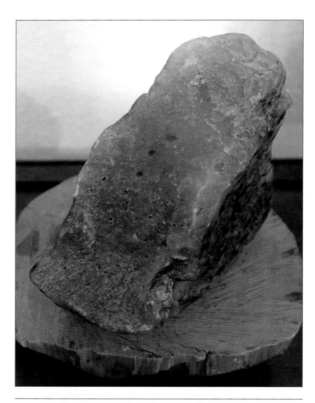

Ambergris, produced in the digestive system of sperm whales, has been highly valued by perfumers as a fixative

Table 17

Top notes	Middle notes	Base notes and fixatives
Bergamot	Caraway	Benzoin
Cinnamon	Cardamom	Cedarwood
Clove	Chamomile	Cistus (fixative)
Lemon	Champaca leaves	Clary sage
Lemongrass	Coriander	Frankincense
Lime	Elemi	Myrrh (fixative)
Neroli	Geranium	Patchouli (fixative)
Orange	Ginger	Peru Balsam
Other citruses	Hyssop	Sandalwood
Peppermint	Lavender and lavandin	Spikenard (fixative)
Petitgrain	Marjoram	Spruce
Thyme	Palmarosa	Vanilla
	Pine	Vetiver (fixative)
	Rosewood	

Oils with More Than One Note

Essential oils have rather complex chemical compositions, which means that many oils have notes in several categories (see fig. 10.2 on the following page). Certain oils even cover the whole spectrum from top note to base note. This is the case of ylang-ylang, jasmine, osmanthus, and tuberose (with a predominance in the middle and base notes) and with champaca flowers and rose (with a predominance in the top and middle notes). Neroli has most of its notes in the top but also has a fair amount of middle notes. It is not surprising that such well-balanced oils are the most pleasant that nature has to offer. They can, in fact, be used by themselves as perfumes.

Blend Equalizers

Blend equalizers are the oils that help you get rid of sharp edges. They fill the gaps, help your blend flow harmoniously, and control the intensity of your most active ingredients.

Most of the blend equalizers are context dependent—they perform better with certain types of blends. Rosewood, champaca flowers, and wild Spanish marjoram are universal equalizers, while orange and tangerine are great with other citruses (neroli, petitgrain, bergamot), spices (clove, cinnamon, nutmeg), and floral fragrances (ylang-ylang, jasmine, rose, geranium). Fir and pine greatly improve blends of Myrtaceae or Coniferae. (See table 18 on page 158.)

The main purpose of blend equalizers is to

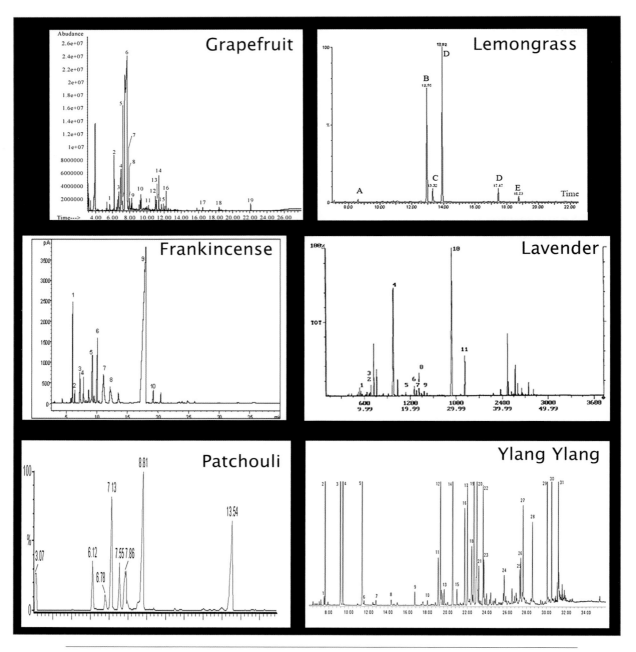

Fig. 10.2. Gas chromatography clearly shows the various subnotes of a particular essential oil. Grapefruit is almost all top to middle notes. Lemongrass is pure middle notes. Frankincense has some middle notes and mostly base notes. Lavender is more complex, with some top notes, lots of middle notes, and some base notes. Patchouli has lots of base notes and fixatives. Ylang-ylang is the most complex, with a full range from top notes to fixatives.

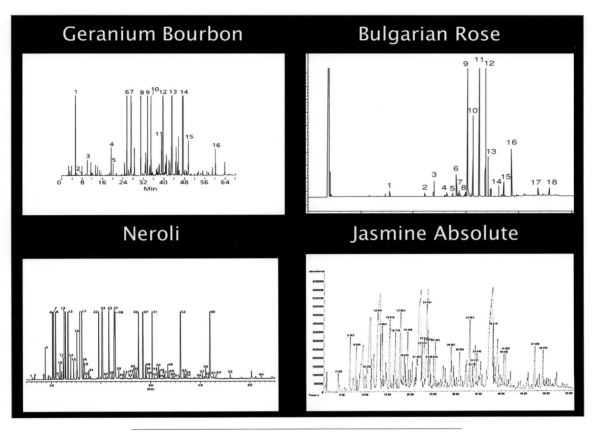

Fig. 10.3. Precious oils typically have a complex structure.

hold your blend together while having little effect on its distinctive personality. They can be used in fairly large amounts (up to 50 percent), especially in those blends where you need to use some of the sharpest oils. Blend equalizers can also be used advantageously with the most precious oils (such as rose, jasmine, neroli, or melissa).

Blend Modifiers (or Personifiers)

Blend modifiers are generally the most intense fragrances. They can greatly affect the overall fragrant quality of your blend, even when used in amounts as small as a fraction of 1 percent.

They are found at each end of the spectrum and are responsible for the sharp edges or deep roots of a blend. They also give your blend its very special kick, contributing to its distinctive personality (but an extra drop or two might kill it). If your blend is rather flat and uninteresting, you can, at your own risk, add such an oil—drop by drop, please!

Typical blend modifiers are clove, cinnamon, peppermint, thyme, blue chamomile, cistus, and patchouli (see table 18 on the following page). Blend modifiers should be used sparingly (never more than 2 to 3 percent).

Table 18

Blend equalizers	Blend modifiers	Blend enhancers	
Champaca leaves	Blue chamomile	Bergamot	Jasmine
Fir	Cinnamon	Cedarwood	Myrrh
Marjoram	Cistus	Champaca flowers	Neroli
Orange	Clove	Clary sage	Osmanthus
Petitgrain	Patchouli	Geranium	Palmarosa
Pine	Peppermint	Lavender	Rose
Rosewood	Thyme	Lemon	Sandalwood
Tangerine		Lime	Spruce
		Litsea cubeba	Ylang-ylang

Blend Enhancers

Between the modifiers and the equalizers we find the enhancers. Enhancers have a pleasant fragrance by themselves. They have enough personality to modify your blend and give it a personal touch, without overpowering it, as long as they are used in reasonable amounts.

Bergamot, cedarwood, geranium, clary sage, lavender, lemon, lime, litsea cubeba, palmarosa, sandalwood, spruce, ylang-ylang and, for the precious oils, jasmine, rose, neroli, and myrrh belong to this category (see table 18). Oils like cajeput, eucalyptus, niaouli, and rosemary could also be considered enhancers, although they are best used in blends for inhalation (diffuser, sauna, steam room, etc.). Enhancers may amount to up to 50 percent of your blend, although each individual oil will rarely account for more than 15 percent of the blend.

Natural Extenders

Some essential oils, such as rose, jasmine, and neroli, are very expensive, and whenever you use them in a blend you want to make sure that their fragrance is not wasted. For instance, I do not recommend blending neroli and red thyme. Red thyme would totally overpower and destroy the neroli. Instead, you want to find essential oils that are as compatible as possible with neroli from an olfactory point of view. Natural extenders are the oils used with the most expensive and precious oils to make affordable blends that respect the notes of the precious oils. (See table 19.)

Further Fragrance Classifications

Many different classifications of fragrances have been created for blending purposes. The most commonly used, in addition to the top, middle, and base notes, is a more descriptive classification

Table 19

Precious oil	Extender
Neroli	Petitgrain, bergamot, tangerine
Rose	Geranium, palmarosa, rosewood
Jasmine	Champaca flowers, ylang-ylang, petitgrain
Champaca flowers	Ylang-ylang, petitgrain
Vanilla	Benzoin, Peru balsam
Sandalwood	Spruce, cedarwood

into floral, fruity, green, balsamic, woody, and so forth. The classification can be refined at will. You may add further notes for your own use.

Here again, many oils are a combination of several notes. For example, lime and lemon are fruity and green. Champaca flower oil has a fruity apricot-like note with a dominance of floral, jasminelike fragrance. Lavender combines floral and herbal. Clary sage is musky and floral. Bergamot is fruity with green and floral notes. Cinnamon is sweet and spicy. Rosemary is herbal and balsamic. The classification here is bound to be highly subjective.

Table 20 describes the most frequently used notes and gives some guidelines to blending proportions as well as to mixing various notes. The oil names in italic are those for which the described note is the dominant note.

Table 20

Note	Blending guidelines	Essential oils
Floral	Usually expensive—the amount to use will be limited by your budget. Blends well with woody, fruity, sweet, vanilla-y, and musky notes, as well as some green notes and some herbal notes. Wasted in balsamic and anise-y notes.	*Rose, neroli, jasmine, ylang-ylang, tuberose, mimosa, osmanthus, champaca flowers, geranium,* palmarosa, lavender, bergamot, petitgrain
Fruity	Inexpensive and easy to blend—can be used in any proportion. Does not blend very well with woods and blends very poorly with balsamics and anise.	*Orange, tangerine, lemon,* lime, grapefruit, bergamot, petitgrain, champaca flowers (apricot note), blue chamomile (apple note)

Table 20 (continued)

Note	Blending guidelines	Essential oils
Green	Blends well with any oil. Use in small amounts (1 to 10 percent), especially the mints.	*Peppermint, spearmint, Mentha arvensis, lime,* lemon, petitgrain, *citronella, lemongrass, Litsea cubeba, melissa, lemon verbena,* bergamot, ginger
Herbal	Blends well with balsamics and woods. Use with caution with flowers.	*Most Labiatae (basil, all sages, hyssop, lavender, marjoram, rosemary, lemon thyme),* angelica, caraway, cardamom, *all chamomiles, coriander, everlasting,* ginger, palmarosa
Balsamic	Gives a very medicinal feel to any blend. Destroys florals. Does not do well with fruits. Best used with woods and herbals.	*Myrtaceae (eucalyptus, niaouli, cajeput, myrtle, tea tree), birch,* cypress, *pine, fir,* rosemary, *spike,* juniper, *terebinth*
Spicy	Use very small amounts (0.5 to 5 percent). Adds an interesting note to any blend. Can also make or break a blend.	*Clove, bay, cinnamon leaf and bark,* nutmeg, pepper, basil eugenol, *oregano, red thyme, savory*
Woody	Blends well with any oil to make the warm, deep heart of the blend (10 to 20 percent).	*Cedarwood, sandalwood, spruce, frankincense,* cypress, juniper
Musky, earthy	Gives depth and roots to any blend. Use in 3 to 10 percent amount.	*Cistus,* clary sage, elemi, *frankincense, myrrh, mugwort, patchouli, vetiver,* angelica
Exotic, sensual	Can be overused. Expensive, but worth every penny. Indulge without excess or may be sickening.	*Jasmine, ylang-ylang, champaca flowers, tuberose, osmanthus, sandalwood, patchouli*
Sweet	Blends with any oils to give warmth and roundness. A fairly large amount of the lighter ones can be used.	*Champaca leaves, marjoram, rosewood,* cardamom, coriander, cinnamon bark, spruce, *tangerine, vanilla, benzoin, Peru balsam*
Anise-y	Difficult to use in blending. Use only in small amounts (10 percent maximum).	*Aniseed, basil, star anise,* caraway, coriander, *fennel, tarragon*
Vanilla-y	Blends with any oil for its characteristic touch but can be overpowering. Use for 2 to 5 percent of blend (maximum 10 percent).	*Vanilla, benzoin, Peru balsam*

Blending Guidelines

Fragrance is a great stimulant of the imagination. Therefore I always encourage people to use images when creating a blend. One of my favorite images for blend creation is that of a human assembly, a social event. Are you coordinating a work group, throwing a lavish party, having a neighborhood barbecue, or preparing for an intimate, romantic evening?

When creating a blend, first look at the purpose of the blend. A blend to fight an infection will be very different from one to soothe emotional wounds or to relieve stress. An infection-fighting blend will be built like a small commando of very efficient no-nonsense soldiers. You want to get the job done, as quickly and cleanly as possible. Your main concern is that the purpose be clear and that all the oils you use work in a very disciplined way toward the same goal. Fragrance is totally secondary.

For emotional problems, on the other hand, fragrance is of the utmost importance, and you will need to carefully and skillfully build your blend to produce a pleasant one. At this level, we can talk about aromatic choreography.

It is important to have a clearly defined purpose when creating a blend. Most beginners try to cure everything with one single blend. Every time I give a seminar on blending, a few students come up with a blend to cure menopause, arthritis, asthma, cellulitis, spleen problems, and stress, plus balance all the chakras in one single shot. This is the best recipe for failure and represents a misunderstanding of the concept of synergy. Essential oils can be used in many ways and applied to many areas of the body. Do not try to treat the lungs and the kidneys with the same blend. Instead, create a blend for each area that you want to address. Create each blend so that it attacks the problem from different angles, treating when possible the causes as well as the symptoms.

Once you determine the purpose of your blend, you have to decide how you are going to use it: through inhalation with a diffuser; applied to the body in massage, bath, compress, or lotion; in skin care preparations; or in special preparations such as personal blends or perfume oils. Lungs are best treated with diffusers or compresses. Emotional issues are best treated with diffusers. Energy issues can be a combination of diffusers and body applications. Physical conditions should be treated through body applications. Be realistic: remember, for example, that inhalation is a useless route for treating cellulite or arthritis.

The more physical the problem, the less important the fragrance of the blend. You should still always try to avoid aromatic disasters. Antiseptic, analgesic, or anticellulite blends need to do the job, whatever it takes. Leave-on blends (lotions, body oils) should be more sophisticated than the take-off blends (bath products, compresses, masks, cleansers). Skin care blends, especially those that are applied at the end of the skin care session (such as toners, creams, and lotions) should have as nice a fragrance as possible—the nose is right in the middle of the face.

Blends for emotional problems should be

as pleasant as possible. For personal blends and perfume oil, sophistication is mandatory. Personal blends are usually created to address deep emotional issues and are used on pressure points and chakras or sniffed directly from the bottle throughout the day. Such blends require a good balance of top, middle, and base notes.

The next step will be to define the theme of the blend, the star of the blend. Are you going to invite a celebrity, such as rose, neroli, jasmine, tuberose, or mimosa, to your gathering? If so, make sure that you don't spoil the party by inviting some rogue oils such as red thyme, savory, clove, or the balsamics. You may use them in very small amounts, just as bodyguards watching the doors, but keep them well under 5 percent. Also, do not invite too many celebrities to the same party. Not only do they run up your bill quite fast, but they also have strong personalities and bicker, or they pout and disappear for the rest of the party. My advice to the beginner is to use the stars only when you really need them and only one at a time, until you figure out who gets along with whom.

Of course, not every blend needs a celebrity. It does not make sense to bring rose or jasmine to treat digestive or intestinal problems. In general, the precious oils are kept for emotional problems or for leave-on types of preparations, especially those applied to the face.

If you choose a celebrity, a precious oil, make sure it is properly surrounded. The entourage should enhance the fragrance of the precious oil. Use the corresponding extenders. Avoid the clashes such as the balsamics with the florals. Use spices sparingly and cautiously. Finally, find a good balance of top, middle, and base. I have found that a small amount of cistus (2 to 4 percent) brings a deep, rich, musk-like base touch to floral blends, especially when combined with 5 to 10 percent of sandalwood.

Precious oils, if treated properly, will add a nice personality to your blend; conversely, without precious oils a blend may lack personality. Blends that use a lot of equalizers (such as marjoram, rosewood, orange, or tangerine), for instance, might end up being rather flat and boring, like a gathering of nice, decent, but rather shy people. Such blends can be greatly enhanced by the modifiers, such as spices and vanilla-y notes.

Unscented Bases and Carrier Oils for Preparations

Once you have mixed your blend, you will use it straight only for inhalation (diffuser, sauna, steam room). For most other purposes, you will need to add some of your blend to a carrier oil or an unscented base. Carrier oils and unscented bases are now readily available; refer to the Resource Guide (unscented products can be purchased by those interested in making their own preparations). Tables 21–35, at the end of this chapter, give proper dosages for the most common preparations.

The Carrier Oils

Many vegetable oils can be used as carriers for your aromatherapy preparations. I classify them into bases and active additives, which will be active ingredients in your preparation. They are used in small amounts for their medicinal and skin rejuvenation or skin protection properties.

The Bases

Apricot kernel oil: A fine and nourishing oil, especially recommended for skin care.

Avocado oil: Used mainly in skin care for its nourishing and restorative properties and its high vitamin content.

Canola oil: Low erucic acid rapeseed oil, expressed from the seeds of *Brassica campestris*. It is very light and odorless and penetrates easily, which makes it a good massage oil base. Its high linoleic acid content prevents rancidity. Low in polyunsaturates, canola oil is good for cooking in that it helps with high cholesterol problems.

Grapeseed oil: The refined oil obtained by pressing numerous varieties of grape seeds. It is a highly polyunsaturated triglyceride oil. A fairly new oil on the American market, it is becoming very popular among beauticians and massage therapists. Very light and odorless, it absorbs easily through the skin. It cleanses, tones, and is widely used in hypoallergenic products as a great emollient film former on skin and hair.

Hazelnut oil: The oil obtained from the nuts of various species of the hazelnut tree, genus *Corylus*. Highly concentrated in vitamin E, it provides deep skin nourishment and moisturizing action and improves cutaneous circulation. It is noncomedogenic and astringent, tightens the pores, and helps normalize sebaceous secretions; therefore it is recommended for oily and combination skin.

Jojoba oil: Expressed or extracted from the bean-like seed of the desert shrub *Simmondsia chinensis*. Used by the Native Americans, jojoba oil is actually a wax; therefore it does not become rancid, which makes it the ideal carrier for perfume oils. Highly emollient, it contains nutrients that feed the skin and regulate its functions. It softens and moisturizes skin, hair, and fingernails. It permeates the stratum corneum, skin, and hair follicles and is very soothing after sun exposure. Some believe that it tends to clog the pores, while others find it very emollient and nourishing for the skin. It is also excellent for hair care (and recommended as a hair oil base).

Sesame oil: Sun protection. Sesamol and sesamoline are natural antioxidants (found only in the virgin cold-pressed oil).

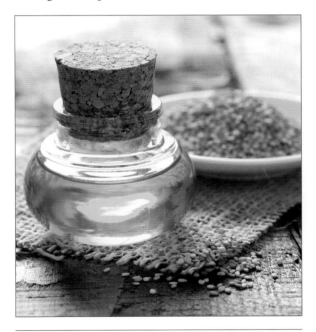

Sesame oil

Sweet almond oil: The triglyceride oil expressed from the ripe seed kernels of the almond tree, Prunus amygdalus dulcis or communis. It is a light, nondrying oil and a natural emollient oil for skin and hair. Since it does not have a good shelf life, keep it in glass and move to smaller containers as the amount you have decreases.

The Active Additives

Squalane: A saturated branched-chain hydrocarbon derived from olives. Occurring naturally in the skin and found in human sebum, it has high affinity with the skin and its natural lipids. It helps the skin act as a barrier and helps avoid transepidermal water loss (TEWL).

Helio-carrot or carrot oil: Obtained from the carrots that are the roots of the *Daucus carota sativa.* Rich in vitamin A, it has cell-regenerating properties. It is recommended before and after sun exposure to help maintain suntan and gives firmness to the skin while helping to prevent wrinkles.

Borage oil: Obtained from the seeds of *Borago officinalis* and very popular in Europe for skin care. It has one of the highest gamma-linolenic acid (GLA) contents (19 to 24 percent). GLA, an essential fatty acid, is at the origin of one class of prostaglandin. It increases the protecting function of skin cells, reinforces the skin as a protecting membrane, and is essential for the function and lipid synthesis of the keratinosomes. Research has demonstrated that GLA applied to the skin is incorporated into phospholipid molecules, which include essential fatty acids known as omega-3 and omega-6 (alpha-linolenic acid). They are essential for health because of their contribution to critical metabolic functions like fingernails, skin, and hair production; visual function; adrenal function (stress); and sperm formation. GLA helps restore the intercellular moisture barrier in the stratum corneum and reduces transepidermal water loss. It moisturizes the skin from within, providing nonocclusive moisturization. Deficiency in GLA increases TEWL, causing severe dryness. Borage oil is recommended in facial oils for its rejuvenative power. It should be refrigerated.

Evening primrose oil: The oil obtained from *Oenothera biennis* or *Oenothera lamarckensi.* It is an expensive oil, rich in gamma-linolenic acid (13 to 15 percent), and therefore excellent for skin care (cf. borage oil). I recommend adding small amounts to a facial oil. This oil, being highly unsaturated, easily becomes rancid and should be refrigerated.

Rosa oil mosqueta: From Chilean rose hip seeds. This is another oil with a high GLA content. It is an emollient, nourishing tissue regenerator and is recommended for facial oils.

Wheat germ oil: Rich in vitamins E, A, and B. Its antioxidant properties make it useful in oil base preparations to prevent rancidity. It helps regenerate tissues and promotes skin elasticity. Being rather heavy and having a fairly strong odor, it is used in small amounts in the carrier.

Vitamin E (tocopherol): An organic heterocyclic compound derived from soy. It protects

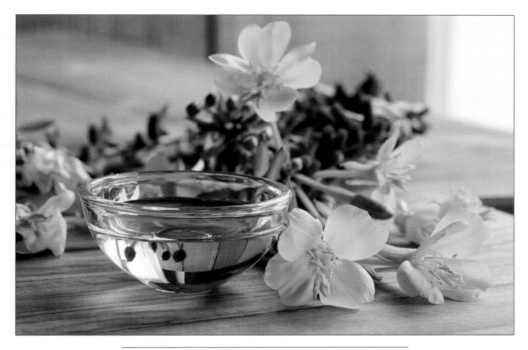

Evening primrose oil

the skin from ultraviolet radiation. It is an excellent natural antioxidant and free-radical scavenger. Free radicals are responsible for the aging process and are caused by numerous environmental factors (pollution, gas pipes, air conditioning, smoking).

Other Carriers: Emulsifiers

Essential oils do not mix directly with water. Emulsifiers are necessary to mix oil and water and therefore needed everytime we want to incorporate essential oils into water. Emulsifiers are molecules with two radicals, one hydrophile (likes water) and one lipophile (likes oil). Several suppliers offer emulsifiers or essential oil solubilizers (see appendix 3).

Suggested base for a facial oil in milliliters (30-milliliter preparation)

Hazelnut oil: 8

Squalene: 8

Jojoba: 8

Helio-carrot: 3

Evening primrose, borage, or *Rosa mosqueta* (or a combination of all): 2

Vitamin E: 1

Suggested base for a massage oil in ounces (4-ounce preparation)

Canola oil: 2

Grapeseed oil: 1.5

Wheat germ oil: 0.5

The Problem of Rancidity

Except for jojoba (which is a wax), any vegetable oil will eventually oxidize and become rancid. Keep your bases in tightly closed dark bottles and store them in a cool place (keep them in your fridge if you use them infrequently). I have noticed that essential oils have antioxidant properties: your aromatherapy preparations will keep longer than the carriers alone. They will have some shelf life but will still eventually go rancid. If stored properly, any oil base preparation should keep for at least six months.

FORMULAS FOR SOME COMMON AILMENTS

Several manufacturers offer an extensive range of premixed blends for a wide range of indications (refer to appendix 3). I encourage you, however, to prepare your own blends. It adds to the fun and the efficiency of your aromatherapy treatment. Tables 21–35 give you some guidelines. Once you become more acquainted with the power of the oils, you will be able to create your own blends.

Table 21
Formulas for Accumulation and Elimination of Toxins and Related Problems

Accumulation and elimination problems		Cellulitis		Obesity and water retention	
Essential Oils	%	Essential Oils	%	Essential Oils	%
Angelica root	5	Birch	10	Birch	10
Birch	20	Cypress	10	Fennel	10
Caraway seeds	5	Fennel	10	Grapefruit	25
Carrot seed	5	Geranium	10	Juniper	10
Coriander seeds	5	Grapefruit	15	Lemon	20
Fennel	15	Lemon	20	Lime	10
Grapefruit	30	Rosemary	20	Orange	10
Juniper	15	Thyme, red	5	Thyme, red	5

Application methods: Bath, compress, massage, friction/unguent, body wrap
Complementary treatments: Drink a lot of liquids (herbal teas or water), including one glass first thing in the morning
Cut down on meat, carbohydrates, milk products, and salt
Eat a lot of raw or steamed vegetables (especially roots)
Exercise
Cellulitis: Massage, frictions, cold showers
Obesity: Emotional support or psychotherapy might be necessary
Build up self-esteem; be good to yourself

Table 22
The Female Cycle

Amenorrhea, dysmenorrhea		Female reproductive system (regulation)		Frigidity	
Essential Oils	*%*	*Essential Oils*	*%*	*Essential Oils*	*%*
Chamomile, German	10	Chamomile, German	5	Clary sage	5
Chamomile, Roman	10	Chamomile, Roman	5	Jasmine	10
Clary sage	15	Clary sage	5	Rose	10
Fennel	10	Fennel	5	Sandalwood	10
Lavender	25	Lavender	35	Tangerine	45
Marjoram	20	Marjoram	40	Ylang-ylang	20
Mugwort	10	Rose	5		

Menopause		Premenstrual syndrome	
Essential Oils	*%*	*Essential Oils*	*%*
Bergamot	20	Carrot seed	5
Chamomile, German	5	Clary sage	10
Chamomile, Roman	5	Fennel	10
Geranium	10	Lavender	20
Jasmine	5	Marjoram	30
Lavender	25	Mugwort	5
Mugwort	5	Rosewood	20
Sage	5		
Ylang-ylang	20		

Application methods: Bath, compress, massage, friction/unguent, douche

Table 23
Articular and Muscular Problems

Arthritis		Muscular and articular pain		Rheumatism	
Essential Oils	*%*	*Essential Oils*	*%*	*Essential Oils*	*%*
Birch	30	Bay	5	Birch	20
Gingerroot	10	Birch	40	Cajeput	10
Juniper	10	Clove buds	5	Gingerroot	10
Marjoram	20	Nutmeg	10	Juniper	10
Rosemary	20	Oregano	5	Marjoram	20
Thyme, red	5	Pepper	5	Nutmeg	10
Vetiver	5	Peppermint	20	Pepper	5
		Rosemary	10	Rosemary	10
				Thyme, red	5

Application methods: Bath, compress, massage, poultice, friction/unguent
Complementary treatments: Drink a lot of liquids (herbal tea and water)
Eat raw and steamed vegetables (celery, cabbage, roots); cut down on salt
Massage and baths are particularly indicated
Moderate exercise

Table 24
Respiratory-Related Disorders

Bronchitis		Colds		Respiratory deficiency	
Essential Oils	*%*	*Essential Oils*	*%*	*Essential Oils*	*%*
Eucalyptus	30	Eucalyptus	20	Cajeput	20
Fir	20	Lavender	20	Eucalyptus	20
Hyssop	10	Pine	20	Fir	20
Lavender	10	Spruce	20	Lavender	20
Myrtle	10	Terebinth	20	Niaouli	10
Pine	10			Peppermint	10
Spruce	10				

Respiratory weakness		Sinusitis	
Essential Oils	*%*	*Essential Oils*	*%*
Fir	40	Eucalyptus	40
Pine	40	Lavender	40
Spruce	30	Peppermint	20

Application methods: Diffuser, compress, massage, friction/unguent
Complementary treatments: Breathing exercises, walks in forest or along beaches
Cut down on carbohydrates and dairy products

Table 25
Blood Circulation

Bruises		Circulation (varicosis, cold feet, tired legs)	
Essential Oils	*%*	*Essential Oils*	*%*
Chamomile, blue	10	Benzoin resinoid	15
Everlasting	20	Cinnamon leaf	5
Geranium	20	Cypress	20
Lavender	50	Geranium	20
		Lemon	30
		Oregano	10

Application methods (bruises): Compress, lotion, friction/unguent
Application methods (circulation): Bath, compress, massage, friction/unguent, body wrap

Table 26
Digestion

Digestive system		Fatigue, anemia, convalescence	
Essential Oils	*%*	*Essential Oils*	*%*
Bergamot	10	Basil	10
Caraway seeds	5	Cardamom	10
Cardamom	5	Gingerroot	10
Coriander seeds	5	Juniper	5
Fennel	5	Nutmeg	10
Gingerroot	5	Peppermint	10
Grapefruit	20	Rosemary	30
Lemon	25	Spearmint	15
Orange	20		
Tangerine	20		

Application methods (digestive): Bath, massage, diffuser, friction/unguent
Application methods (fatigue, etc.): Bath, diffuser, massage, friction/unguent

Table 27
Headaches and Migraines

Headaches		Migraines		Digestive origin of migraines	
Essential Oils	%	Essential Oils	%	Essential Oils	%
Chamomile, Roman	10	Lavender	30	Basil	10
Lavender	20	Marjoram	30	Chamomile, Roman	10
Peppermint	20	Melissa	10	Gingerroot	10
Rosewood	40	Peppermint	20	Lavender	20
Spearmint	10	Spearmint	10	Marjoram	30
				Peppermint	20
				Spearmint	10

Application methods: Compress, diffuser, massage, friction/unguent
Complementary treatments: Relaxation, breathing exercises
Avoid heavy food (meat, eggs, rich sauces, etc)
Physical exercise

Table 28
Impotence

Eastern blend		Spicy blend	
Essential Oils	%	Essential Oils	%
Champaca leaves	20	Clary sage	10
Cistus	5	Gingerroot	10
Clary sage	10	Nutmeg	10
Jasmine	20	Pepper	10
Sandalwood, Mysore	20	Peppermint	10
Vetiver	5	Sandalwood, Mysore	20
Ylang-ylang	20	Vetiver	10
		Ylang-ylang	20

Application methods: Bath, compress, massage, friction/unguent
Complementary treatments: Relaxation; exercise; avoid stress
Eat proteins and spicy, earthy food (meat may be recommended)
Avoid alcohol excess

Table 29
Infectious Diseases and Epidemics

Essential Oils	%
Eucalyptus	30
Lavender	20
Myrtle	20
Peppermint	10
Tea tree	10
Thyme, red	10

Application methods: Bath, compress, diffuser, massage, friction/unguent

Table 30
Insect Repellents

Fleas		Mosquitos		Moths	
Essential Oils	%	Essential Oils	%	Essential Oils	%
Lavandin	30	Citronella	25	Lavandin	50
Lavender	30	Geranium	25	Lavender	50
Pennyroyal	20	Lemongrass	25		
Spike	20	Pennyroyal	25		

Application methods (fleas): Diffuser, friction/unguent, sprinkle in infested areas

Application methods (mosquitos): Diffuser, lotion, friction/unguent

Application methods (moths): Diffuser, place an aromatic pottery in a drawer

Table 31
Insomnia

Essential Oils	%	Essential Oils	%
Chamomile, Roman	10	Marjoram	20
Lavender	20	Neroli	20
Marjoram	20	Orange	15
Orange	15	Spikenard	10
Spikenard	10	Tangerine	15
Tangerine	15	Ylang-ylang	20
Ylang-ylang	10		

Application methods: Baths, diffuser, massage
Complementary treatments: Relaxation, yoga, breathing exercise
Physical exercise (work out)
Avoid stress
Balance your diet; vitamins and minerals are advised

Table 32
Emotional Problems, Stress, and Brain Stimulation

Anxiety		Depression			
		Indulging formula		Uplifting formula	
Essential Oils	%	Essential Oils	%	Essential Oils	%
Benzoin resinoid	10	Bergamot	10	Lemon	10
Bergamot	10	Geranium	15	Lime	20
Clary sage	10	Jasmine	10	Melissa	10
Jasmine	10	Petitgrain	10	Peppermint	10
Lemon	10	Rose	5	Petitgrain	20
Patchouli	10	Rosewood	20	Rosemary	20
Petitgrain	20	Sandalwood, Mysore	10	Thyme, lemon	10
Rosewood	20	Ylang-ylang	20		

Application methods: Baths, diffuser, massage
Complementary treatments: Relax, be good to yourself, treat yourself
Start a new project
Physical exercise is strongly recommended
Balance your diet; vitamins and minerals are suggested

Table 32 *(continued)*

Emotional shock, grief		Neurasthenia		Sadness	
Essential Oils	*%*	*Essential Oils*	*%*	*Essential Oils*	*%*
Melissa	10	Lavender	20	Benzoin resinoid	20
Neroli	10	Melissa	10	Jasmine	10
Rose	10	Patchouli	10	Rose	10
Sandalwood	10	Rosemary	40	Rosewood	40
Tangerine	60	Thyme, lemon	20	Ylang-ylang	20

Application methods: Baths, diffuser, massage
Complementary treatments: Yoga, meditation
Psychotherapy and emotional support are strongly advised

Energy		Memory (poor)		Mental fatigue	
Essential Oils	*%*	*Essential Oils*	*%*	*Essential Oils*	*%*
Benzoin resinoid	10	Basil	10	Basil	20
Cedarwood	20	Clove buds	10	Cardamom	20
Clary sage	10	Gingerroot	10	Gingerroot	20
Fir	30	Juniper	10	Peppermint	20
Spruce	30	Petitgrain	30	Rosemary	20
		Rosemary	30		

Application methods: Baths, diffuser, massage
Complementary treatments: Take vitamins and minerals
Reduce stress
Balance diet (eat enough protein)

Nervous tension, nervousness		Stress		Tension	
Essential Oils	*%*	*Essential Oils*	*%*	*Essential Oils*	*%*
Geranium	10	Cedarwood	20	Clary sage	20
Lavender	10	Clary sage	20	Lavender	20
Marjoram	20	Fir	20	Marjoram	20
Melissa	10	Pine	20	Petitgrain	20
Neroli	10	Spruce	20	Ylang-ylang	20
Tangerine	40	Ylang-ylang	20		
Ylang-ylang	10				

Application methods: Baths, diffuser, massage
Complementary treatments: Relaxation (yoga or meditation)
Massage and baths are strongly recommended

Table 33
Skin Care Formulas

Acne		Dermatitis		Wrinkles	
Essential Oils	*%*	*Essential Oils*	*%*	*Essential Oils*	*%*
Bergamot	10	Cedarwood	10	Clary sage	5
Juniper	5	Juniper	5	Frankincense	5
Lavender	10	Lavender	10	Geranium	20
Palmarosa	20	Litsea cubeba	10	Myrrh	5
Peppermint	5	Palmarosa	20	Patchouli	5
Rosemary	10	Peppermint	10	Rose	10
Sandalwood, Mysore	10	Rosewood	20	Rosemary	20
Thyme, lemon	30	Thyme, lemon	15	Rosewood	30

Dry skin		Oily skin		Sensitive skin	
Essential Oils	*%*	*Essential Oils*	*%*	*Essential Oils*	*%*
Clary sage	10	Clary sage	10	Chamomile, Roman	5
Jasmine	10	Frankincense	10	Everlasting	5
Palmarosa	30	Geranium	20	Jasmine	10
Rose	10	Lavender	10	Neroli	10
Rosemary	20	Lemon	30	Rose	10
Sandalwood	20	Ylang-ylang	20	Rosewood	60

Application methods: Facials, masks, compresses, lotions, facial and body oils, body wraps

Table 34
Hair Care Formulas

Oily hair		Hair loss (growth)		Dandruff	
Essential Oils	*%*	*Essential Oils*	*%*	*Essential Oils*	*%*
Cedarwood	25	Bay	20	Cedarwood	20
Lemongrass	25	Cedarwood	20	Patchouli	20
Rosemary	25	Clary sage	10	Rosemary	20
Sage	25	Rosemary	20	Sage	20
		Sage	10	Tea tree	20
		Ylang-ylang	20		

Application methods: Shampoos, rinses, conditioners, hair oils

Table 35
Chakra and Energy Formulas

Crown chakra		Third eye		Heart chakra	
Essential Oils	*%*	*Essential Oils*	*%*	*Essential Oils*	*%*
Benzoin resinoid	10	Cistus	5	Benzoin resinoid	40
Cistus	5	Frankincense	5	Melissa	10
Frankincense	5	Mugwort	10	Neroli	30
Myrrh	10	Myrrh	10	Rose	20
Rose	10	Sandalwood, Mysore	20		
Sandalwood, Mysore	20	Spruce	50		
Spruce	40				

Solar plexus		Sacral chakra		Root chakra	
Essential Oils	*%*	*Essential Oils*	*%*	*Essential Oils*	*%*
Clove	10	Jasmine	20	Frankincense	30
Juniper	10	Sandalwood	20	Pepper	40
Lemon	30	Tangerine	30	Vetiver	30
Rosemary	30	Ylang-ylang	30		
Sage	20				

Yoga, meditation, rituals		Astral bodies		Psychic centers	
Essential Oils	*%*	*Essential Oils*	*%*	*Essential Oils*	*%*
Cedarwood	20	Lavender	20	Cedarwood	25
Cistus	5	Marjoram	30	Cistus	5
Fir	30	Melissa	10	Elemi	10
Myrrh	5	Patchouli	10	Frankincense	10
Sandalwood, Mysore	15	Rosemary	20	Myrrh	10
Spruce	25	Thyme, lemon	10	Spruce	40

Application methods: Unguent, diffuser, massage

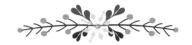

Essential Oils
Reference Table

This table has been created to help you find rapidly the information that you may need in your daily practice. It might seem overwhelming at first glance, but I hope you find it comprehensive and practical. Many oils listed here cannot be found easily in any other book. I also differentiate between the varieties of the same species (such as chamomiles or the chemotypes of thyme). Since there are a few hundred essential oils, some have been left out. Still, I cover all the common oils plus all those that present some therapeutic interest and can be found on the market.

The following codes represent suggested uses of oils for specific conditions:

D   Diffuser
M   Massage
B   Bath
F   Facial masks
C   Compresses
L   Lotions
O   Oil for face or body
U   Unguents

The power of the oil is indicated with regard to the specific condition on a scale from 1 to 5.

Plant name (*Genus species/family*)	Property	Indication	Use	Power
Angelica root (*Angelica archangelica*/ Umbelliferae)	Medicinal			
	Cleanser, depurative, drainer	Accumulation (toxins, fluids)	MBFCLO	4
	Stimulant digestive	Digestive problems, migraine	DCU	3
	Revitalizing, stimulant	Anemia, asthenia, anorexia convalescence, rachitism	DMB	4
	Carminative	Aerophagia	MBC	3
	Cleanser, depurative, drainer	Gout	MCU	3
	Antispasmodic	Digestive spasms	MBCU	3
Aniseed (*Pimpinella anisum*/ Umbelliferae)	Medicinal			
	Carminative	Aerophagia	MBC	4
	Digestive stimulant	Digestive problems, migraine	DCU	4
	Antispasmodic	Digestive spasms	MBCU	3
	Galactagogue	Insufficient milk	MBCU	3
	Aphrodisiac	Frigidity, impotence	MBCU	2
Basil (*Ocimum basilicum*/ Lamiaceae)	Medicinal			
	Antiseptic (intestinal)	Intestinal infections	MCU	3
	Stimulant	Vital centers	DMBU	4
	Cephalic	Migraine	DCU	4
	Antispasmodic, stomachic	Dyspepsia, gastric spasms	MCU	3
	Facilitates birth and nursing	Nursing, pregnancy	DMBU	2
	Mind, emotion, psyche			
	Stimulant	Memory (poor), neurovegetative system	DMBU	4
	Tonic (nervous)	Nervous fatigue, intellectual, mental fatigue, mental strain	DMBU	4
	Contraindications			
	Stupefying	High doses	D	2
Bay (*Pimenta racemosa*/ Myrtaceae)	Body and skin care			
	Scalp stimulant	Hair growth	LO	4
	Medicinal			
	Antiseptic, stimulant	Respiratory system	DMBU	3
	Antiseptic	Infectious diseases	DMBU	3
	Analgesic, antineuralgic	Pain (muscular and articular), neuralgia	MBCU	3

Plant name (*Genus species/ family*)	Property	Indication	Use	Power
Benzoin resinoid (*Styrax benzoin/* Styraceae)	<u>Body and skin care</u>			
	Rejuvenating, stimulant	Skin elasticity	FCLOU	2
	<u>Medicinal</u>			
	Appeasing, balancing	Energy inbalance	DMB	4
	Regulator	Secretions	MBCU	3
	Expectorant	Bronchitis	DMBC	3
	Soothing	Cough, laryngitis	D	3
	Stimulant	Circulation	MBCU	2
	Antiseptic, diuretic	Genitourinary infections, urinary infections	MBC	2
	Healing	Cracked and chapped skin, dermatitis, skin irritation, skin rashes, wounds	CLU	4
	<u>Mind, emotion, psyche</u>			
	Purifier	Drive out evil spirits	DU	3
	Stimulant	Crown chakra, heart chakra	DU	3
	Comforting, euphoric	Anxiety, loneliness, sadness	DMBU	3
	Comforting, uplifting	Exhaustion (psychic and emotional)	DMBU	3
Bergamot (*Citrus bergamia/* Rutaceae)	<u>Body and skin care</u>			
	Antiseptic, vulnerary	Acne, eczema, seborrhea	FCLO	3
	<u>Medicinal</u>			
	Refreshing	Hot climates	DMBLU	3
	Stimulant	Digestive problems	MBC	3
	Balancing	Nervous system	DMBU	4
	Antispasmodic, digestive	Colics, intestinal infections	MCU	3
	Antiseptic, vulnerary	Leukorrhea, vaginal pruritus	MU	3
	<u>Mind, emotion, psyche</u>			
	Antidepressant, uplifting	Anxiety, depression	DMB	4
	<u>Contraindications</u>			
	Increases photosensitivity	Do not apply neat before sun exposure	MFCLOU	3

Plant name (*Genus species/ family*)	Property	Indication	Use	Power
Birch (*Betula lenta* and *betula nigra*/ Betulaceae)	<u>Medicinal</u>			
	Analgesic	Arthritis, pain (muscular and articular), rheumatism	MBCU	4
	Cleanser, depurative, drainer	Accumulation (toxins, fluids), cellulitis, obesity, water retention	MBCU	3
	Diuretic	Cystitis, kidneys	MBCU	4
Cajeput (*Melaleuca leucadendra*/ Myrtaceae)	<u>Medicinal</u>			
	Balancing, re-equilibrating	Energy inbalance	DMB	3
	Antiseptic, antispasmodic	Respiratory system	DMBCU	5
	Antiseptic	Infectious diseases	DMBCU	4
	Antiseptic (urinary)	Cystitis, urethritis, urinary infections	MBC	4
	Balsamic, expectorant	Asthma, bronchitis, tuberculosis	DMBCU	5
	Antineuralgic	Rheumatism	MBCU	3
	Antiseptic (intestinal)	Amoebas, diarrhea, dysentery	MB	3
	Analgesic, antiseptic	Earache	U	4
	Antiseptic, expectorant	Sinusitis	DU	5
Caraway seeds (*Carum carvi*/ Umbelliferae)	<u>Medicinal</u>			
	Cleanser, depurative, drainer	Accumulation (toxins, fluids)	MBFCLO	3
	Stimulant, digestive stimulant	Digestive problems	MBC	4
	Stimulant general	Energy deficiency	DMB	3
	Carminative	Aerophagia, fermentation	MBC	4
	Antispasmodic	Dyspepsia, migraine, digestive spasms	MBCU	3
	Parasiticide	Scabies	CLU	2
	Diuretic	Kidneys	MBCU	2
	Tissue regenerator	Infected wounds	FCLOU	3
	Stimulant	Glandular system	MBU	2
	<u>Mind, emotion, psyche</u>			
	Tonic (nervous)	Mental fatigue, mental strain	DMBU	3

Plant name (*Genus species*/family)	Property	Indication	Use	Power
Cardamom (*Eletteria cardamomum*/ Zingiberaceae)	Medicinal			
	Stimulant	Digestive problems	MBC	4
	Aphrodisiac	Impotence	MBCU	3
	Antidiarrheal	Diarrhea	MBCU	3
Carrot seed (*Daucus carota*/ Umbelliferae)	Body and skin care			
	Cleanser, depurative, drainer	Dermatitis	MFCLOU	3
	Stimulate elasticity, tonic	Aged skin, skin irritation, skin rashes, wrinkles	FCLO	3
	Medicinal			
	Cleanser, depurative, drainer	Accumulation (toxins, fluids)	MBFCLO	4
	Stimulant general	Energy deficiency	DMB	2
	Revitalizing, stimulant	Anemia, asthenia, anorexia, convalescence, rachitism	DMB	3
	Cleanser, depurative, hepatic	Hepatobiliary disorders	MBCU	4
	Emmenagogue	Amenorrhea, dysmenorrhea, premenstrual syndrome	MBCU	3
	Stimulant	Glandular system	MBU	3
Chamomile, blue (*Ormensis multicaulis*/ Asteraceae)	Body and skin care			
	Anti-inflammatory, soothing	Acne, dermatitis, eczema, skin care	FCLO	5
	Anti-inflammatory, soothing	Inflamed skin, sensitive skin	FCLO	4
	Medicinal			
	Analgesic, anti-inflammatory	Arthritis, inflamed joints	BCU	4
	Anti-inflammatory, healing, soothing	Abscess, boils, bruises	CLU	4
	Antispasmodic, sedative	Colics, colitis	MBC	3
	Cholagogue, hepatic	Liver and spleen congestion	MCU	3
	Analgesic, anti-inflammatory	Teething pain, toothache	U	3
Chamomile, German (*Chamomilla matricaria*/ Asteraceae)	Body and skin care			
	Anti-inflammatory, soothing	Acne, dermatitis, eczema, skin care	FCLO	3
	Anti-inflammatory, soothing	Inflamed skin, sensitive skin	FCLO	4

Plant name (*Genus species/ family*)	Property	Indication	Use	Power
	Medicinal			
	Immunostimulant	Leukocyte formation stimulant	DMU	4
	Analgesic, anti-inflammatory	Arthritis, inflamed joints	BCU	4
	Anti-inflammatory, healing, soothing	Abscess, boils	FCLO	4
	Antispasmodic, sedative	Colics, colitis	MCU	4
	Calming, sedative	Headache, insomnia, irritability, migraine	DCU	4
	Emmenagogue	Amenorrhea, dysmenorrhea, menopause	DMBCU	4
	Analgesic	Teething pain, toothache	U	4
	Antianemic	Anemia, asthenia	DMB	4
	Digestive, stomachic	Digestive problems	MBC	4
	Cholagogue, hepatic	Liver, liver and spleen congestion	MCU	4
	Balancing	Female reproductive system	DMBCU	4
	Mind, emotion, psyche			
	Appeasing	Anger, tantrum	DMBU	4
Chamomile, mixta (*Anthemis mixta/* Asteraceae)	Body and skin care			
	Calming, soothing	Sensitive skin	FCLO	4
	Medicinal			
	Antispasmodic, sedative	Colic, colitis	MCU	3
	Calming, sedative	Headache, insomnia, irritability, migraine	DCU	3
	Emmenagogue	Amenorrhea, dysmenorrhea, menopause	DMBCU	3
	Cholagogue, hepatic	Liver and spleen congestion	MCU	3
Chamomile, Roman (*Anthemis nobilis/* Asteraceae)	Body and skin care			
	Healing, soothing	Abscess, boils, sensitive skin	FCLO	5
	Medicinal			
	Analgesic	Arthritis, inflamed joints	BCU	3
	Antispasmodic, sedative	Colic, colitis	MCU	4
	Calming, sedative	Headache, insomnia, irritability, migraine	DCU	4

Plant name (*Genus species/family*)	Property	Indication	Use	Power
	Emmenagogue	Amenorrhea, dysmenorrhea, menopause	DMBCU	4
	Analgesic	Teething pain, toothache	U	4
	Antianemic	Anemia, asthenia	DMB	4
	Digestive, stomachic	Digestive problems	MBC	4
	Immunostimulant	Leukocyte formation stimulant	DMU	4
	Cholagogue, hepatic	Liver, liver and spleen congestion	MCU	4
	Balancing	Female reproductive system	DMBCU	4
	Mind, emotion, psyche			
	Realization	Personal growth	DMBU	4
	Appeasing	Anger, oversensitivity, tantrum	DMBU	4
Cedarwood (*Cedrus atlantica/* Coniferae)	Body and skin care			
	Antiseptic, fungicidal	Dandruff, hair loss	LO	4
	Antiseborrheic	Oily hair	LO	3
	Medicinal			
	Tonic	Glandular system, nervous system, respiratory system	DMBCU	4
	Antiseptic (urinary)	Cystitis, urinary infections	MBC	3
	Antiseptic, fungicidal	Dermatitis, eczema, fungal infections, ulcers	FCLO	4
	Mind, emotion, psyche			
	Appeasing	Deep relaxation	DMBU	4
	Appeasing, sedative	Anxiety, stress	DMB	3
	Elevating, grounding, opening	Psychic work, yoga, meditation, rituals	DU	3
Cinnamon bark (*Cinnamomum zeylanicum/* Lauraceae)	Medicinal			
	Stimulant	Circulation, heart, nervous system	DMBU	4
	Antiseptic	Flu, infectious diseases	DMBCU	5
	Antispasmodic	Spasms	DMBC	2
	Stimulant	Anemia, asthenia, digestive problems	MBC	3

Plant name (*Genus species*/family)	Property	Indication	Use	Power
	Parasiticide	Lice, scabies	CLU	3
	Aphrodisiac	Impotence	MBCU	2
	Antiseptic	Intestinal infections	MCU	3
	Contractions stimulant	Childbirth	MCU	3
	Contraindications			
	Irritant (skin)	High doses, neat or in high concentration	BFC	3
	Convulsive	High doses		3
Cinnamon leaf (*Cinnamomum zeylanicum*/Lauraceae)	Medicinal			
	Stimulant	Circulation	MBCU	4
	Antiseptic	Infectious diseases	DMBCU	5
	Parasiticide	Lice, scabies	CLU	3
	Antiseptic	Intestinal infections	MCU	3
	Contraindications			
	Irritant (skin)	High doses, neat or in high concentration	BFC	4
	Convulsive	High doses		4
Cistus (*Cistus ladanifer*/Cistaceae)	Medicinal			
	Diuretic	Urinary infections	MBC	3
	Drying, vulnerary	Ulcers, wounds	CLU	2
	Mind, emotion, psyche			
	Stimulant	Third eye, crown chakra	DU	5
	Stimulant	Psychic centers	DU	5
	Sedative (nervous)	Insomnia, nervousness	DMBU	3
	Elevating, grounding, opening	Psychic work, yoga, meditation, rituals	DU	5
Citronella (*Cymbopogon nardus*/Poaceae)	Medicinal			
	Deodorant, deodorizer, purifier	Sanitation, epidemics	D	4
	Insect repellent	Mosquitos	DLU	5
	Deodorant, deodorizer	Bathroom, garbage	D	4
	Stimulant	Digestive problems	MBC	2
	Antiseptic	Infectious diseases	DMBCU	3

Plant name (*Genus species/family*)	Property	Indication	Use	Power
Clary sage (*Salvia sclarea/* Lamiaceae)	Body and skin care			
	Cell regenerator	Aged skin, wrinkles	FCLO	3
	Soothing	Inflamed skin	FCLO	3
	Regulator of seborrhea	Dry skin, oily skin	FCLO	3
	Regulator of seborrhea	Oily skin	LO	3
	Scalp stimulant, stimulant	Hair growth	LO	3
	Medicinal			
	Antispasmodic, emmenagogue	Menstrual cramps, premenstrual syndrome	MBCU	4
	Emmenagogue	Amenorrhea, dysmenorrhea	MBCU	4
	Balancing, tonic	Female reproductive system, feminine energy	DMBU	5
	Mind, emotion, psyche			
	Antidepressant, calming	Anxiety, emotional tension, stress, tension	DMBU	2
	Antidepressant, euphoric	Depression, postnatal depression	DMB	4
Clove buds (*Eugenia caryophyllata/* Myrtaceae)	Medicinal			
	Antiseptic, stimulant	Respiratory system	DMBCU	5
	Antiseptic	Infectious diseases	DMBCU	4
	Antiseptic (urinary)	Urinary infections	MBC	4
	Analgesic, antineuralgic	Pain (muscular and articular), neuralgia, toothache	U	5
	Carminative, stomachic	Dyspepsia, fermentations	MBC	4
	Stimulant	Anemia, asthenia, energy deficiency	DMB	4
	Aphrodisiac	Impotence	MBCU	3
	Antiseptic, cicatrizant	Infected wounds, ulcers	FCLO	3
	Parasiticide	Scabies	CLU	3
	Mind, emotion, psyche			
	Stimulant (intellectual)	Nervous fatigue, intellectual, memory (poor)	DMBU	4

Plant name (*Genus species/family*)	Property	Indication	Use	Power
Coriander seeds (*Coriandrum sativum/* Umbelliferae)	Medicinal			
	Cleanser, depurative, drainer	Accumulation (toxins, fluids)	MBFCLO	3
	Stimulant, digestive	Digestive problems	MBC	4
	Revitalizing, stimulant	Anemia, asthenia, convalescence	DMB	4
	Carminative	Aerophagia, flatulence	MBCU	4
	Analgesic, warming	Gout, rheumatism	MBCU	3
	Aperitive, revitalizing	Anorexia	DMB	3
	Antispasmodic	Migraine, digestive spasms	MBCU	3
	Stimulant	Glandular system	MBU	3
Cumin seeds (*Cuminum cymimum* Umbelliferae)	Medicinal			
	Cleanser, depurative, drainer	Accumulation (toxins, fluids)	MBFCLO	3
	Revitalizing, stimulant	Anemia, asthenia, convalescence	DMB	3
	Carminative	Aerophagia, flatulence	MBCU	4
	Antispasmodic	Digestive spasms	MBCU	3
	Digestive	Digestive problems, migraine	DCU	3
	Stimulant	Heart, nervous system	DMBU	3
Cypress, (*Cupressus sempervirens/* Coniferae)	Medicinal			
	Warming	Energy deficiency	DMB	4
	Tonic	Respiratory system	DMBCU	3
	Tonic (circulation)	Cellulitis, circulation	MBCU	5
	Astringent	Edema, water retention	MBCU	5
	Antispasmodic	Asthma, cough, whooping cough	DMC	4
	Antisudorific, deodorant, deodorizer	Perspiration (especially of feet)	MBCLU	4
Elemi (*Canarium luzonicum/* Burseraceae)	Medicinal			
	Cooling, drying, vulnerary	Infected wounds	FCLOU	3
	Regulator	Secretions	MBCU	4
	Balsamic, expectorant	Catarrhal condition	D	2
	Balsamic	Respiratory system	DMBCU	2
	Mind, emotion, psyche			
	Fortifying	Psychic centers	DU	3

Plant name (*Genus species/* family)	Property	Indication	Use	Power
Eucalyptus australiana, *Eucalyptus polybractea* (Myrtaceae)	Medicinal			
	Balancing, re-equilibrating	Energy inbalance	DMB	4
	Antiseptic, stimulant	Respiratory system	DMBCU	5
	Antiseptic	Infectious diseases	DMBCU	4
	Antiseptic (urinary)	Urinary infections	MBC	4
	Balsamic, expectorant	Asthma, bronchitis tuberculosis	DMBCU	5
	Antidiabetic	Diabetes	MB	3
	Antiseptic, expectorant	Sinusitis	DU	5
Eucalyptus citriodora (Myrtaceae)	Medicinal			
	Antiseptic, bactericidal	Infectious diseases	DMBCU	3
	Deodorant, deodorizer, disinfectant	Sanitation	D	3
Eucalyptus globulus (Myrtaceae)	Medicinal			
	Balancing, re-equilibrating	Energy inbalance	DMB	4
	Antiseptic, stimulant	Respiratory system	DMBCU	5
	Antiseptic	Infectious diseases	DMBCU	4
	Antiseptic (urinary)	Urinary infections	MBC	4
	Balsamic, expectorant	Asthma, bronchitis, tuberculosis	DMBCU	5
	Vermifuge	Ascarides, oxyurids	MBCU	3
	Antidiabetic	Diabetes	MB	3
Everlasting (*Helichrysum italicum/* Asteraceae)	Body and skin care			
	Anti-inflammatory, soothing	Acne, dermatitis, skin care	FCLO	3
	Anti-inflammatory, soothing	Inflamed skin, sensitive skin	FCLO	4
	Anti-inflammatory, astringent, healing	Hemorrhage, skin irritation	FCLOU	5
	Medicinal			
	Anti-inflammatory, healing, soothing	Abscess, boils	FCLO	4
	Tissue stimulant	Wounds, cuts	CLU	5
	Cholagogue, hepatic	Liver, liver and spleen congestion	MCU	4

Plant name (*Genus species/family*)	Property	Indication	Use	Power
Fennel (*Foeniculum vulgare/* Umbelliferae)	Body and skin care			
	Cleanser, detoxifier	Orange-peel skin	MBCU	5
	Medicinal			
	Cleanser, depurative, drainer	Accumulation (toxins, fluids)	MBFCLO	5
	Stimulant, stimulant digestive	Digestive problems	MBC	4
	Revitalizing, stimulant	Anemia, asthenia, rachitism	DMB	4
	Carminative	Aerophagia, flatulence	MBCU	3
	Antispasmodic	Digestive spasms	MBCU	3
	Cleanser, detoxifier	Cellulitis, obesity, orange-peel skin, water retention	MBCU	5
	Regulator	Amenorrhea, dysmenorrhea, female reproductive system, premenstrual syndrome	MBCU	4
	Galactagogue	Insufficient milk (nursing), nursing	DMBU	4
	Stimulant	Glandular system, glandular system (estrogen)	MBU	4
	Contraindications			
	Toxic	Young children (under 6)	MBU	2
Fir (*Abies balsamea/* Coniferae)	Medicinal			
	Warming	Respiratory weakness	DMBU	4
	Tonic	Glandular system, nervous system, respiratory system	DMBCU	4
	Antiseptic (urinary)	Genitourinary infections, urinary infections	MBC	3
	Antiseptic, expectorant	Asthma, bronchitis	DMBC	4
	Mind, emotion, psyche			
	Elevating, grounding, opening	Psychic work	DU	5
	Elevating, grounding, opening	Third eye, crown chakra	DU	5
	Appeasing, sedative	Anxiety stress	DMB	5
	Elevating, grounding, opening	Yoga, meditation, rituals	DU	5

Plant name (*Genus species/family*)	Property	Indication	Use	Power
Frankincense (*Boswellia carterii/* Burseraceae)	Body and skin care			
	Revitalizing, tonic	Aged skin, wrinkles	FCLO	4
	Medicinal			
	Cooling, drying, vulnerary	Infected wounds, inflammations	FCLU	4
	Regulator	Secretions	MBCU	4
	Balsamic, expectorant	Asthma, catarrhal condition, cough	D	3
	Antiseptic (pulmonary)	Lungs	DCU	3
	Mind, emotion, psyche			
	Fortifying	Mind, psychic centers	DU	5
	Stimulant	Third eye, crown chakra	DU	4
Geranium (*Pelargonium graveolens* and *roseum/* Geraniaceae)	Body and skin care			
	Antiseptic, astringent, cell regenerator	Acne, aged skin, dermatitis, oily skin, skin care	FCLO	3
	Medicinal			
	Astringent, hemostatic	Bruises, hemorrhage	CLU	4
	Antiseptic	Infectious diseases	DMBCU	3
	Antidiabetic	Diabetes	MB	3
	Diuretic	Kidney stones, kidneys	MBCU	3
	Adrenal cortex stimulant	Cellulitis, adrenocortical glands, menopause	DMBCU	3
	Insect repellent	Mosquitos	DLU	3
	Astringent	Sore throat, tonsillitis	U	3
	Antiseptic, cytophilactic	Burns, wounds	CLU	3
	Mind, emotion, psyche			
	Stimulant, uplifting	Depression, nervous tension	DMBU	3
Gingerroot (*Zingiber officinale/* Zingiberaceae)	Medicinal			
	Stimulant	Digestive problems, memory (poor), neurovegetative system, vital centers	DMBU	4
	Stimulant	Digestive problems	MBC	3
	Cephalic	Migraine	DCU	3
	Antispasmodic, stomachic	Dyspepsia, gastric spasms	MCU	3
	Analgesic	Arthritis, rheumatism	MBCU	3

Plant name (*Genus species*/ family)	Property	Indication	Use	Power
	Febrifuge	Fever	MBCU	3
	Carminative	Aerophagia, flatulence	MBCU	3
	Aphrodisiac	Impotence	MBCU	3
	Antidiarrheal	Diarrhea	MBCU	3
	Antiseptic, astringent	Sore throat, tonsillitis	U	3
	Mind, emotion, psyche			
	Stimulant	Memory (poor)	DMBU	4
Grapefruit (*Citrus paradisi*/ Rutaceae)	Medicinal			
	Stimulant	Digestive problems	MBC	3
	Control of liquid processes	Lymphatic system and secretions, secretions	MBCU	5
	Drainer, lymphatic stimulant	Cellulitis, obesity, water retention	MBCU	5
Hyssop (*Hyssopus officinalis*/ Lamiaceae)	Medicinal			
	Stimulant	Respiratory system, vital centers	DMBU	4
	Antispasmodic, balsamic, expectorant	Asthma, bronchitis, catarrhal condition, whooping cough	DMC	5
	Antispasmodic, expectorant	Whooping cough	DMC	5
	Hypertensor	Hypotension	DMCU	4
	Digestive, stomachic	Digestive problems, dyspepsia	MCU	3
	Cicatrizant, vulnerary	Dermatitis, eczema, wounds	CLU	2
Jasmine (*Jasminum officinalis*/ Oleaceae)	Body and skin care			
	Moisturizer, soothing	Dry skin, sensitive skin	FCLO	3
	Healing, soothing	Dermatitis	MFCLOU	3
	Medicinal			
	Aphrodisiac	Frigidity, impotence	MBCU	5
	Mind, emotion, psyche			
	Stimulant	Sexual chakra	DMBU	5
	Antidepressant, euphoric	Anxiety, lethargy, menopause, sadness	DMBU	5
	Uplifting	Lack of confidence	DMBU	4
	Antidepressant, euphoric	Depression, postnatal depression	DMB	5

Plant name (*Genus species/ family*)	Property	Indication	Use	Power
Juniper (*Juniperus communis/* Coniferae)	Body and skin care			
	Cleanser, detoxifier, drainer	Acne, dermatitis, eczema	FCLO	4
	Medicinal			
	Tonic	Glandular system	MBU	4
	Antiseptic (urinary)	Genitourinary infections, urinary infections	MBC	5
	Diuretic, urinary antiseptic	Cystitis, diabetes, oliguria	MBCU	4
	Cleanser, detoxifier, drainer	Accumulation (toxins, fluids), arthritis, rheumatism, uric acid	MBCU	5
	Mind, emotion, psyche			
	Tonic (nervous)	Nervous and intellectual fatigue, memory (poor)	DMBU	4
Lavender (*Lavandula officinalis/* Lamiaceae)	Body and skin care			
	Antiseptic, cytophilactic	Acne, dermatitis, eczema, oily skin	FCLO	4
	Healing	Psoriasis	CLU	3
	Medicinal			
	Stimulant	Metabolism, respiratory system, vital centers	DMBU	4
	Antiseptic	Blennorrhea, cystitis, infectious diseases	DMBCU	5
	Antiseptic, cytophylactic	Abscess, bruises, burns, wounds	CLU	5
	Antiseptic, antispasmodic	Asthma, bronchitis, catarrhal condition, colds	DMCU	4
	Decongestant	Sinusitis	DU	5
	Calming, cephalic	Headache, migraine	DCU	4
	Calming	Insomnia, nervous tension, palpitations	DMBC	3
	Insect repellent	Fleas, moths	DU	3
	Antispasmodic, emmenagogue	Amenorrhea, dismenorrhea, menopause, premenstrual syndrome	MBCU	3
	Mind, emotion, psyche			
	Appeasing	Astral body	DMBU	4
	Antidepressant, calming	Depression, neaurasthenia	DMB	4
	Anticonvulsive	Convulsions	DMBC	4

Plant name (*Genus species/family*)	Property	Indication	Use	Power
Lavandin (*Lavandula fragrans* and *delphinensis*/ Lamiaceae)	Medicinal			
	Stimulant	Respiratory system	DMBCU	3
	Antiseptic	Infectious diseases	DMBCU	4
	Antiseptic, cytophilactic	Burns, wounds	CLU	3
	Deodorant, deodorizer, disinfectant	Sanitation, epidemics	D	3
	Insect repellent	Fleas, mosquitos	DLU	3
	Mind, emotion, psyche			
	Appeasing	Astral body	DMBU	3
Lemon (*Citrus limon*/ Rutaceae)	Body and skin care			
	Antiseptic, depurative, lymphatic stimulant	Oily skin, skin care	FCLO	4
	Medicinal			
	Digestive, stimulant	Digestive problems	MBC	4
	Control of liquid processes	Lymphatic system and secretions, secretions	MBCU	4
	Hepatobiliary stimulant	Gallbladder congestion, liver	MCU	4
	Tonic	Nervous system	DMBU	4
	Antiseptic, immunostimulant	Infectious diseases, viral diseases	DMU	4
	Immunostimulant	Leukocyte formation stimulant	DMU	5
	Stimulant, tonic, uplifting	Anemia, asthenia, convalescence	DMB	4
	Blood fluidifier, hypotensive	Hypertension, hyperviscosity	MBU	4
	Antivirus	Herpes, immune system (low)	DMB	3
	Drainer, lymphatic stimulant	Cellulitis, obesity, water retention	MBCU	4
	Mind, emotion, psyche			
	Antidepressant, uplifting	Anxiety, depression	DMB	4
Lemongrass (*Cymbopogon citratus*/ Poaceae)	Body and skin care			
	Astringent, tonic	Open pores	FCLO	3
	Medicinal			
	Deodorant, deodorizer, disinfectant	Sanitation	D	3
	Insect repellent	Mosquitos	DLU	2

Plant name (*Genus species*/ family)	Property	Indication	Use	Power
	Stimulant	Digestive problems	MBC	3
	Digestive, stomachic	Digestive problems	MBC	3
	Regulator	Parasympathic system	DMB	3
	Antiseptic	Infectious diseases	DMBCU	3
	Contraindications			
	Irritant (skin)	Neat or in high concentration	MBFCLOU	2
Lime (*Citrus aurantifolia*/ Rutaceae)	Medicinal			
	Refreshing	Hot climates	DMBLU	4
	Digestive, stimulant	Digestive problems	MBC	4
	Control of liquid processes	Lymphatic system and secretions, secretions	MBCU	3
	Hepatobiliary stimulant	Gallbladder congestion, liver	MCU	4
	Tonic	Nervous system	DMBU	4
	Stimulant, tonic, uplifting	Anemia, asthenia, convalescence	DMB	3
	Drainer, lymphatic stimulant	Obesity, water retention	MBCU	3
	Antiseptic, antispasmodic	Asthma, bronchitis, catarrhal condition	D	3
	Mind, emotion, psyche			
	Antidepressant, uplifting	Anxiety, depression	DMB	4
Litsea cubeba (Poaceae)	Body and skin care			
	Healing, soothing	Dermatitis	MFCLOU	3
	Medicinal			
	Deodorant, deodorizer, disinfectant	Sanitation, epidemics	D	3
	Stimulant	Digestive problems	MBC	3
Lovage root (*Levisticum officinale*/ Umbelliferae)	Medicinal			
	Cleanser, depurative, drainer	Accumulation (toxins, fluids)	MBFCLO	3
	Stimulant, digestive stimulant	Digestive problems, intestines	MBC	3
	Stimulant	Kidneys	MBCU	3
	Revitalizing, stimulant	Anemia, asthenia	DMB	3
	Carminative	Aerophagy, flatulence	MBCU	3

Plant name (*Genus species*/family)	Property	Indication	Use	Power
	Cleanser, depurative, drainer	Gout, rheumatism	MBCU	2
	Antispasmodic	Digestive spasms	MBCU	2
	Diuretic	Cystitis, albuminuria	MBCU	4
	Emmenagogue	Amenorrhea, dysmenorrhea	MBCU	3
	Diuretic	Edema, urine retention, water retention	MBCU	3
Marjoram, wild Spanish (*Thymus mastichina*/ Lamiaceae)	Medicinal			
	Calming	Respiratory system	DMBCU	2
	Antispasmodic	Spasms digestive, spasms respiratory	DMCU	4
	Analgesic, sedative	Migraine	DCU	4
	Analgesic, sedative	Arthritis, rheumatism	MBCU	3
	Mind, emotion, psyche			
	Calming, sedative	Insomnia, nervous tension	DMBU	3
Marjoram (*Origanum marjorana* and *Marjorana hortensis*/ Lamiaceae)	Medicinal			
	Antispasmodic	Digestive spasms, respiratory spasms	DMBU	4
	Antispasmodic, emmenagogue	Amenorrhea, dysmenorrhea, premenstrual syndrome	MBCU	3
	Hypotensor, vasodilator	Hypertension	MBU	4
	Analgesic, sedative	Migraine	DCU	4
	Analgesic, sedative	Arthritis, rheumatism	MBCU	3
	Antispasmodic, digestive	Dyspepsia, flatulence	MBCU	2
	Mind, emotion, psyche			
	Appeasing	Astral body	DMBU	4
	Calming, sedative	Insomnia, nervous tension tension	DMBU	4
Melissa (*Melissa officinalis*/ Lamiaceae)	Body and skin care			
	Antiseptic, cytophilactic	Acne, dermatitis, eczema	FCLO	3
	Medicinal			
	Stimulant	Metabolism, vital centers	DMBU	4
	Antivirus	Viral diseases	DMU	4
	Calming, sedative	Insomnia, migraine, nervous tension	DMBC	4

Plant name (*Genus species/family*)	Property	Indication	Use	Power
	Mind, emotion, psyche			
	Appeasing	Astral body	DMBU	4
	Antidepressant, calming	Depression, neurasthenia	DMB	5
	Stimulant	Heart chakra	DU	5
	Appeasing, soothing, uplifting	Emotional shock, grief	DMBU	5
Mugwort (*Artemisia vulgaris/* Asteraceae)	Medicinal			
	Emmenagogue	Amenorrhea, dysmenorrhea, menopause, premenstrual syndrome	MBCU	5
	Analgesic	Teething pain, toothache	U	4
	Balancing	Female reproductive system	DMBCU	5
	Cholagogue	Hepatobiliary disorders	MBCU	3
	Vermifuge	Ascaris, oxyurides	MMBU	3
	Mind, emotion, psyche			
	Opening	Dream, psychic work	DU	5
	Contraindications			
	Abortive	Pregnancy	DMBU	4
Myrrh (*Commiphora myrrha/* Burseraccae)	Body and skin care			
	Revitalizing, tonic	Aged skin, wrinkles	FCLO	4
	Medicinal			
	Cooling, drying	Inflammations	FCLU	4
	Regulator	Secretions	MBCU	4
	Balsamic, expectorant	Asthma, catarrhal condition, cough	D	4
	Antiseptic (pulmonary)	Lungs	DUC	3
	Cooling, drying, vulnerary	Infected wounds	FCLOU	4
	Fungicidal	Thrush	Douche	4
	Antiseptic, astringent	Cough, mouth ulcers and inflammations, sore throat	U	4
	Mind, emotion, psyche			
	Fortifying	Mind, psychic centers	DU	5
	Stimulant	Third eye, crown chakra	DU	4

Plant name (*Genus species/* family)	Property	Indication	Use	Power
Myrtle (*Myrtus communis/* Myrtaceae)	Medicinal			
	Balancing, re-equilibrating	Energy imbalance	DMB	4
	Antiseptic, stimulant	Respiratory system	DMBCU	5
	Antiseptic	Infectious diseases	DMBCU	4
	Antiseptic (urinary)	Urinary infections	MBC	4
	Balsamic, expectorant	Asthma, bronchitis, tuberculosis	DMBCU	5
Neroli (*Citrus aurantium* blossom Rutaceae)	Body and skin care			
	Soothing	Sensitive skin	FCLO	5
	Medicinal			
	Hypotensor, sedative	Palpitations	DMBC	3
	Mind, emotion, psyche			
	Sedative	Hysteria, insomnia, nervous tension, nervousness	DMBU	5
	Antidepressant, sedative	Emotional shock, grief	DMBU	5
	Stimulant	Heart chakra	DU	5
Niaouli (*Melaleuca viridiflora/* Myrtaceae)	Medicinal			
	Balancing, re-equilibrating	Energy imbalance	DMB	4
	Antiseptic, stimulant	Respiratory system	DMBCU	5
	Antiseptic	Infectious diseases	DMBCU	4
	Antiseptic (urinary)	Urinary infections	MBC	4
	Balsamic, expectorant	Asthma, bronchitis, tuberculosis	DMBCU	5
	Tissue stimulant	Acne, burns, wounds	CLU	4
	Anticatarrhal	Catarrhal condition	D	5
	Antiseptic, expectorant	Sinusitis	DU	5
Nutmeg (*Myristica fragrans/* Myristicaceae)	Medicinal			
	Stimulant	Digestive problems	MBC	4
	Analgesic	Pain (muscular and articular), neuralgia, rheumatism	MBCU	3
	Aphrodisiac	Impotence	MBCU	3
	Carminative	Flatulence	MBCU	3
	Antiseptic	Intestines	MBC	3

Plant name (*Genus species*/family)	Property	Indication	Use	Power
	Mind, emotion, psyche			
	Stimulant	Nervous and intellectual fatigue	DMB	3
	Contraindications			
	Stupefying, toxic	High doses	D	3
Orange, sweet (*Citrus aurantium*/Rutaceae)	Medicinal			
	Digestive, stimulant	Digestive problems	MBC	3
	Control of liquid processes	Lymphatic system and secretions, secretions	MBCU	2
	Drainer, lymphatic stimulant	Obesity, water retention	MBCU	3
	Hypotensor, sedative	Palpitations	DMBC	2
	Digestive, stimulant	Digestive problems	MBC	3
	Mind, emotion, psyche			
	Sedative	Hysteria, insomnia, nervous tension	DMBU	3
Oregano (*Origanum vulgare*/Lamiaceae)	Medicinal			
	Stimulant	Metabolism, respiratory system, vital centers	DMBU	4
	Stimulant	Metabolism	DMBU	4
	Stimulant	Respiratory system	DMBCU	4
	Antitoxic, antivirus	Viral diseases	DMU	5
	Antiseptic, cytophilactic	Abscess, burns, wounds	CLU	3
	Antiseptic, antispasmodic	Asthma, bronchitis, catarrhal condition	D	3
	Antiseptic, antitoxic	Infectious diseases	DMBCU	3
	Antiseptic	Blennorrhea, cystitis	MBCU	3
	Revulsive, rubefacient	Circulation, pain (muscular and articular), circulation (capillary)	MBCLOU	4
	Contraindications			
	Irritant (skin)	Neat or in high concentration	FC	4

Plant name (*Genus species/ family*)	Property	Indication	Use	Power
Palmarosa (*Cymbopogon martinii/* Poaceae)	Body and skin care			
	Antiseptic, cell regenerator	Acne, dermatitis, skin care	FCLO	3
	Antiseptic, cell regenerator stimulant	Skin care, general skin care	FCLO	3
	Moisturizer, soothing	Dry skin	FCLO	3
	Medicinal			
	Stimulant	Digestive problems	MBC	3
Patchouli (*Pogostemon patchouli/* Lamiaceae)	Body and skin care			
	Antiphlogistic, regenerator	Acne, dermatitis, eczema	FCLO	4
	Tissue regenerator	Aged skin, cracked and chapped skin, wrinkles	FCLO	4
	Fungicidal, tissue regenerator	Impetigo	FCL	3
	Regulator	Seborrhea	FCLO	3
	Decongestant	Skin care	FCLO	3
	Medicinal			
	Fungicidal	Dandruff, fungal infections	CLU	4
	Mind, emotion, psyche			
	Appeasing	Astral body	DMBU	4
	Antidepressant, calming	Anxiety, neurasthenia	DMB	4
Pennyroyal (*Mentha pulegium/* Lamiaceae)	Medicinal			
	Digestive, stomachic	Dyspepsia, gastralgia, nausea, vomiting	MCU	4
	Emmenagogue	Amenorrhea, dysmenorrhea	MBCU	4
	Insect repellent	Fleas, mosquitos	DLU	4
	Contraindications			
	Abortive	Pregnancy	DMBU	5
	Toxic	Ingestion	D	3
Pepper (*Piper nigrum/* Piperaceae)	Medicinal			
	Stimulant	Digestive problems, nervous system	DMBU	3
	Aphrodisiac	Impotence	MBCU	3
	Antitoxic	Food poisoning	MU	3
	Digestive, stomachic	Dyspepsia	MCU	3
	Analgesic, rubefacient	Pain (muscular and articular), neuralgia, rheumatism	MBCU	3
	Febrifuge	Fever	MBCU	2

Plant name (*Genus species*/ family)	Property	Indication	Use	Power
	Mind, emotion, psyche			
	Stimulant	Root chakra	MU	3
	Comforting	Ungroundedness	DMBU	3
Peppermint (*Mentha piperita*/ Lamiaceae)	Body and skin care			
	Cleanser, decongestant	Acne, dermatitis	MFCLOU	4
	Medicinal			
	Stimulant	Metabolism, nervous system, respiratory system, vital centers	DMBU	4
	Antiseptic	Infectious diseases	DMBCU	3
	Antiseptic, antispasmodic	Asthma, bronchitis, catarrhal condition	D	3
	Decongestant	Sinusitis	DU	4
	Calming, cephalic	Headache, migraine	DCU	4
	Stimulant (nervous system)	Fainting, vertigo	DC	4
	Digestive, stomachic	Dyspepsia, gastralgia, nausea, vomiting	MCU	5
	Cholagogue, hepatic	Hepatobiliary disorders	MBCU	4
	Febrifuge	Fever	MBCU	4
	Aphrodisiac	Impotence	MBCU	4
	Analgesic, antineuralgic	Pain (muscular and articular), neuralgia	MBCU	4
	Mind, emotion, psyche			
	Antidepressant, tonic	Depression, neurasthenia	DMB	4
	Stimulant (nervous system)	Fatigue, mental fatigue, mental strain	DMBU	5
Petitgrain biguarade (*Citrus aurantium* leaf/ Rutaceae)	Medicinal			
	Digestive, stimulant	Digestive problems	MBC	3
	Antispasmodic, digestive	Dyspepsia, flatulence	MBCU	3
	Mind, emotion, psyche			
	Clarifying, refreshing	Confusion	DMBU	4
	Antidepressant, uplifting	Anxiety, depression	DMB	3
	Stimulant, tonic	Memory (poor), mental fatigue, mental strain, nervous system	DMBU	4

Plant name (*Genus species*/ family)	Property	Indication	Use	Power
Pine (*Pinus sylvestris*/ Coniferae)	Medicinal			
	Warming	Respiratory weakness	DMBU	3
	Tonic	Glandular system, nervous system, respiratory system	DMBCU	3
	Antiseptic (urinary)		MBC	3
		Genitourinary infections, urinary infections	U	4
	Expectorant, pectoral	Colds, sore throat		
	Mind, emotion, psyche		DMB	3
	Appeasing, sedative	Anxiety, stress		
Rose (*Rosa centifolia* and *damascena*/ Rosaceae)	Body and skin care			
	Cell regenerator	Aged skin, eczema, sensitive skin, wrinkles	FCLO	5
	Moisturizer	Dry skin	FCLO	4
	Medicinal			
	Regulator	Female reproductive system	DMBCU	4
	Aphrodisiac	Frigidity, impotence	MBCU	4
	Astringent, hemostatic	Hemorrhage	CLU	3
	Mind, emotion, psyche			
	Stimulant	Heart chakra	DU	5
	Uplifting	Emotional shock, grief	DMBU	5
	Antidepressant, uplifting	Depression, nervous tension, sadness	DMBU	5
Rosemary (*Rosmarinus officinalis*/ Lamiaceae)	Body and skin care			
	Antiseptic, cytophilactic	Acne, dermatitis, eczema	FCLO	4
	Regulator of seborrhea	Dry skin	FCLO	3
	Rejuvenating	Aged skin, wrinkles	FCLO	4
	Regulator, scalp stimulant	Dandruff, hair loss, oily hair	LO	4
	Medicinal			
	Antiseptic, cytophilactic	Abscess, burns, wounds	CLU	3
	Antiseptic, antispasmodic	Asthma, bronchitis, catarrhal condition	D	3
	Stimulant	Adrenocortical glands, metabolism, respiratory system, vital centers	DMBU	4

Plant name (*Genus species/ family*)	Property	Indication	Use	Power
	Tonic	Anemia, asthenia, debility	DMB	4
	Stimulant (hepatobiliary)	Cholecystitis, cirrhosis, gallbladder congestion, hangover, jaundice	DMBCU	4
	Cardiotonic	Heart	DMBU	3
	Analgesic, rubefacient	Arthritis, pain (muscular and articular)	MCU	3
	Mind, emotion, psyche			
	Appeasing	Astral body	DMBU	4
	Antidepressant, uplifting	Depression, neurasthenia	DMB	4
	Tonic (nervous)	Memory (poor), mental fatigue, mental strain	DMBU	4
Rosewood (*Aniba roseaodora/* Lauraceae)	Body and skin care			
	Antiseptic, cell regenerator	Acne, dermatitis, skin care	FCLO	5
	Cell regenerator, regenerator	Aged skin, sensitive skin, wrinkles	FCLO	5
	Medicinal			
	Calming, cephalic	Headache, nausea	DMCU	4
	Mind, emotion, psyche			
	Antidepressant, uplifting	Anxiety, sadness	DMBU	4
Sage (*Salvia officinalis* and *lavandulifolia/* Lamiaceae)	Body and skin care			
	Depurative, healing	Acne, dermatitis, eczema	FCLO	4
	Regulator of seborrhea	Dandruff, hair loss	LO	4
	Medicinal			
	Stimulant	Adrenocortical glands, metabolism, nervous system, vital centers	DMBU	4
	Stimulant	Metabolism	DMBU	4
	Stimulant	Nervous system	DMBU	4
	Stimulant	Adrenocortical glands	MB	4
	Tonic	Anemia, asthenia, debility	DMB	4
	Stimulant (hepatobiliary)	Cholecystitis, jaundice	DMBCU	4
	Hypertensor	Hypotension	DMCU	4
	Emmenagogue	Amenorrhea, dysmenorrhea, menopause, sterility	MBCU	4
	Antisudorific	Sweating (excessive)	MBCLU	
	Mind, emotion, psyche			4
	Antidepressant, uplifting	Depression, neurasthenia	DMB	4
	Tonic (nervous)	Fatigue, mental fatigue, mental strain	DMBU	4

Plant name (*Genus species*/ family)	Property	Indication	Use	Power
	Contraindications			
	Abortive, toxic	High doses	MBCU	4
Sandalwood, Mysore (*Santalum album*/ Santalaceae)	Body and skin care			
	Healing, moisturizer, soothing	Acne, cracked and chapped skin, dry skin	FCLO	3
	Medicinal			
	Antiseptic (urinary)	Blennorrhea, cystitis, gonorrhea	LU	3
	Mind, emotion, psyche			
	Elevating, grounding, opening	Third eye, crown chakra	DU	4
	Elevating, grounding, opening	Yoga, meditation, rituals	DU	5
	Antidepressant, euphoric	Depression	DMB	3
Savory (*Satureja montana*/ Lamiaceae)	Medicinal			
	Stimulant	Nervous system	DMBU	4
	Antibiotic, antiseptic	Infectious diseases	DMBCU	5
	Tonic	Anemia, asthenia, debility	DMB	4
	Analgesic, rubefacient	Arthritis, rheumatism	MBCU	4
	Contraindications			
	Irritant (skin)	Neat or in high concentration	BFC	4
Spearmint (*Mentha viridis*/ Lamiaceae)	Body and skin care			
	Cleanser, decongestant	Acne, dermatitis	MFCLOU	3
	Medicinal			
	Decongestant	Sinusitis	DU	3
	Stimulant	Metabolism, nervous system, respiratory system, vital centers	DMBU	3
	Antiseptic, antispasmodic	Asthma, bronchitis, catarrhal condition	D	3
	Calming, cephalic	Headache, migraine	DCU	3

Plant name (*Genus species*/ family)	Property	Indication	Use	Power
	Digestive, stomachic	Dyspepsia, nausea, vomiting	MCU	4
	Digestive, stomachic	Dyspepsia, gastralgia	MCU	4
	Cholagogue, hepatic	Hepatobiliary disorders	MBCU	4
	Febrifuge	Fever	MBCU	2
	Mind, emotion, psyche			
	Antidepressant, tonic	Depression, neurasthenia	DMB	4
	Stimulant (nervous system)	Fatigue, mental fatigue, mental strain	DMBU	3
Spike (*Lavandula spica*/ Lamiaceae)	Medicinal			
	Stimulant	Respiratory system	DMBCU	3
	Insect repellent	Fleas	DU	4
	Analgesic, rubefacient	Pain (muscular and articular), sport preparation	MCU	4
	Antiseptic, cytophilactic	Abscess, burns, wounds	CLU	3
Spruce (*Picea mariana*/ Coniferae)	Medicinal			
	Tonic	Glandular system, nervous system, respiratory system	DMBCU	3
	Warming	Respiratory weakness	DMBU	5
	Antiseptic, expectorant	Asthma, bronchitis	DMBC	4
	Mind, emotion, psyche			
	Elevating, grounding, opening	Psychic work	DU	5
	Elevating, grounding, opening	Third eye, crown chakra	DU	5
	Appeasing, sedative	Anxiety, stress	DMB	5
	Elevating, grounding, opening	Yoga, meditation, rituals	DU	5
Tangerine (*Citrus reticulata*/ Rutaceae)	Medicinal			
	Digestive, stimulant	Digestive problems	MBC	3
	Control of liquid processes	Lymphatic system and secretions, secretions	MBCU	2
	Antispasmodic, digestive	Dyspepsia, flatulence	MBCU	3
	Drainer, lymphatic stimulant	Obesity, water retention	MBCU	2
	Mind, emotion, psyche			
	Sedative	Hysteria, insomnia, nervous tension, nervousness	DMBU	3
	Sedative, soothing	Emotional shock, grief	DMBU	2

Plant name (*Genus species*/ family)	Property	Indication	Use	Power
Tarragon (*Artemisia dracunculus*/ Asteraceae)	Medicinal			
	Antispasmodic, digestive	Digestive and intestinal spasms, dyspepsia, hiccup	MCU	4
	Carminative	Aerophagia, fermentation	MBC	4
	Vermifuge	Ascarides, oxyurids	MBCU	3
Tea tree (*Melaleuca alternifolia*/ Myrtaceae)	Body and skin care			
	Cicatrizant, fungicidal, vulnerary	Abscess, acne, herpes, pruritis, skin irritation, skin rashes	FCLOU	4
	Fungicidal	Dandruff, hair care	LO	4
	Medicinal			
	Antiseptic, stimulant	Respiratory system	DMBCU	5
	Antiinfectious	Infectious diseases	DMBCU	4
	Antiseptic (urinary)	Urinary infections	MBC	4
	Balsamic, expectorant	Asthma, bronchitis, tuberculosis	DMBCU	5
	Fungicidal	Athlete's foot, *Candida*, fungal infections, ringworm, vaginitis	CLOU	5
	Antiinfectious	Infected wounds, sores	CLOU	4
Terebinth (*Pinus maritimus*/ Coniferae)	Medicinal			
	Tonic	Glandular system, respiratory system	DMBCU	3
	Antiseptic (urinary)	Genitourinary infections, urinary infections	MBC	4
	Antiseptic, expectorant	Asthma, bronchitis	DMBC	4
	Expectorant, pectoral	Colds, sore throat	U	4
	Antiseptic, expectorant	Asthma, bronchitis	DMBC	4
Thyme, hyemalis (*Thymus hyemalis*/ Lamiaceae)	Body and skin care			
	Healing, soothing	Acne, dermatitis, eczema	FCLO	4
	Medicinal			
	Stimulant	Metabolism, vital centers	DMBU	4
	Antibiotic, antiseptic	Infectious diseases	DMBCU	3
	Antiseptic, cytophilactic	Abscess, burns, wounds	CLU	3
	Calming	Insomnia, palpitations	DMBC	3
	Mind, emotion, psyche			
	Antidepressant, uplifting	Depression, neurasthenia	DMB	3

Plant name (*Genus species*/ family)	Property	Indication	Use	Power
Thyme, lemon (*Thymus citriodorus*/ Lamiaceae)	<u>Medicinal</u>			
	Stimulant	Metabolism, nervous system, vital centers	DMBU	4
	Antibiotic, antiseptic	Infectious diseases	DMBCU	3
	Antiseptic, cytophilactic	Abscess, burns, wounds	CLU	3
	Antiseptic, antispasmodic	Asthma, bronchitis, catarrhal condition	D	3
	Tonic	Anemia, asthenia, debility	DMB	3
	<u>Mind, emotion, psyche</u>			
	Appeasing	Astral body	DMBU	4
	Antidepressant, uplifting	Depression, neurasthenia	DMB	4
Thyme, red (*Thymus zygis*/ Lamiaceae)	<u>Medicinal</u>			
	Stimulant	Metabolism, vital centers	DMBU	4
	Antibiotic, antiseptic	Infectious diseases	DMBCU	5
	Antiseptic (intestinal)	Intestinal infections	MCU	5
	Antiseptic (urinary)	Blennorrhea, cystitis	MBCU	3
	Tonic	Anemia, asthenia, debility	DMB	3
	Analgesic, rubefacient	Arthritis, circulation (capillary), rheumatism, sport preparation	MCU	4
	Stimulant circulation capillary	Cellulitis, circulation, obesity	MBCLOU	3
	Stimulant, uplifting	Depression, neurasthenia	DMB	3
	<u>Contraindications</u>			
	Irritant (skin)	Neat or in high concentration	BFC	4
Verbena, lemon (*Lippia citriodora*/ Verbenaceae)	<u>Medicinal</u>			
	Hepatobiliary stimulant	Liver	MCU	3
	Calming	Tachycardia	DMBCU	3
	<u>Mind, emotion, psyche</u>			
	Regulator	Neurovegetative system	DMBU	3
	Calming	Nervousness	DMBU	3
Vetiver (*Andropogon muricatus*/ Poaceae)	<u>Medicinal</u>			
	Rubefacient	Arthritis	MBCU	4
	<u>Mind, emotion, psyche</u>			
	Stimulant	Root chakra	MU	4
	Comforting	Ungroundedness	DMBU	4

Plant name (*Genus species*/family)	Property	Indication	Use	Power
Ylang-ylang (*Unona odoratissima*/Anonaceae)	Body and skin care			
	Antiseborrheic	Oily skin	FCLO	3
	Scalp stimulant	Hair growth	LO	3
	Medicinal			
	Hypotensive	Hyperpnea, hypertension, palpitations, tachycardia	DMBCU	4
	Aphrodisiac	Frigidity, impotence	MBCU	4
	Mind, emotion, psyche			
	Antidepressant, euphoric	Depression, menopause, stress	DMB	3
	Sedative	Insomnia, nervous tension	DMBU	3
	Stimulant	Sexual chakra	DMBU	3
	Calming, euphoric	Anger, fear, frustration	DMBU	3

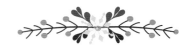

Aromatherapy Therapeutic Index

BEAUTY, SKIN, AND HAIR CARE

Acne

Bergamot, blue chamomile, German chamomile, everlasting, geranium, juniper, lavender, melissa, niaouli, palmarosa, patchouli, peppermint, rosemary, rosewood, Spanish sage, Mysore sandalwood, spearmint, tea tree, lemon thyme
Application methods: Compress, facial, mask, lotion, face oil/body oil

Aged Skin

Carrot seed, clary sage, frankincense, geranium, myrrh, patchouli, rose, rosemary, rosewood
Application methods: Compress, facial, mask, lotion, face oil/body oil, body wrap

Cracked and Chapped Skin

Benzoin resinoid, patchouli, Mysore sandalwood
Application methods: Compress, facial, mask, lotion, friction/unguent

Dandruff

Cedarwood, patchouli, rosemary, Spanish sage, tea tree
Application methods: Lotion, hair oil, shampoo

Dermatitis

Benzoin resinoid, blue chamomile, German chamomile, carrot seed, cedarwood, everlasting, geranium, jasmine absolute, juniper, lavender, Litsea cubeba, melissa, palmarosa, patchouli, peppermint, rosemary, rosewood, Spanish sage, spearmint, lemon thyme
Application methods: Compress, facial, mask, lotion, massage, face oil/body oil, friction/unguent

Dry Skin

Clary sage, jasmine absolute, palmarosa, rose, rosemary, Mysore sandalwood
Application methods: Compress, facial, mask, lotion, face oil/body oil

Eczema

Bergamot, blue chamomile, German chamomile, cedarwood, juniper, lavender, melissa, patchouli, rose, rosemary, Spanish sage, lemon thyme
Application methods: Compress, facial, mask, lotion, face oil/body oil

Hair Growth

Bay, clary sage, ylang-ylang
Application methods: Lotion, face oil/body oil, shampoo

Hair Loss

Cedarwood, rosemary, Spanish sage, ylang-ylang
Application methods: Lotion, face oil/body oil, shampoo

Inflamed Skin

Blue chamomile, German chamomile, clary sage, everlasting
Application methods: Compress, facial, mask, lotion, face oil/body oil, body wrap

Oily Hair

Cedarwood, clary sage, rosemary
Application methods: Lotion, face oil/body oil, shampoo

Oily Skin

Clary sage, geranium, lavender, lemon, ylang-ylang
Application methods: Compress, facial, mask, lotion, face oil/body oil

Seborrhea

Bergamot, patchouli, sage

Application methods: Compress, facial, mask, lotion, face oil/body oil, body wrap

Sensitive Skin

Blue chamomile, chamomile mixta, Roman chamomile, German chamomile, everlasting, jasmine absolute, neroli, rose, rosewood
Application methods: Compress, facial, mask, lotion, face oil/body oil, body wrap

Skin Care

Blue chamomile, German chamomile, everlasting, geranium, lemon, palmarosa, patchouli, rosewood
Application methods: Compress, facial, mask, lotion, face oil/body oil, body wrap

Skin Irritation, Skin Rashes

Benzoin resinoid, carrot seed, everlasting, tea tree
Application methods: Compress, facial, mask, lotion, face oil/body oil, friction/unguent

Wrinkles

Carrot seed, clary sage, frankincense, myrrh, patchouli, rose, rosemary, rosewood, spikenard
Application methods: Compress, facial, mask, lotion, face oil/body oil

MEDICINAL INDICATIONS

Abscess

Blue chamomile, Roman chamomile, German chamomile, everlasting, lavender, oregano, rosemary, spike, tea tree, lemon thyme
Application methods: Compress, facial, mask, lotion, face oil/body oil

Accumulation (Toxins, Fluids)

Angelica root, birch, caraway seeds, carrot seed, coriander seeds, cumin seeds, fennel, juniper, lovage root

Application methods: Bath, compress, facials, mask, lotion, massage, face oil/body oil, body wrap

Adrenocortical Glands

Geranium, rosemary, Spanish sage

Application methods: Bath, massage

Aerophagy

Angelica root, aniseed, caraway seeds, cardamom, coriander seeds, cumin seeds, fennel, ginger root, lovage root, tarragon

Application methods: Bath, compress, massage

Amenorrhea, Dysmenorrhea

Chamomile mixta, Roman chamomile, German chamomile, carrot seed, clary sage, fennel, lavender, lovage root, marjoram, mugwort, pennyroyal, Spanish sage

Application methods: Bath, compress, massage, friction/unguent, douche

Anemia, Asthenia

Angelica root, Roman chamomile, German chamomile, carrot seed, cinnamon bark, clove buds, coriander seeds, cumin seeds, fennel, lemon, lime, lovage root, petitgrain biguarade, rosemary, Spanish sage, savory, lemon thyme, red thyme

Application methods: Bath, diffuser, massage

Anorexia

Angelica root, carrot seed, coriander seeds

Application methods: Bath, diffuser, massage

Arthritis

Birch, blue chamomile, Roman chamomile, German chamomile, gingerroot, juniper, marjoram, wild Spanish marjoram, rosemary, savory, red thyme, vetiver

Application methods: Bath, compress, massage, friction/unguent, body wrap

Asthma

Cajeput, cypress, *Eucalyptus australiana, E. globulus,* fir, frankincense, hyssop, lavender, lime, myrrh, myrtle, niaouli, oregano, peppermint, rosemary, spearmint, spruce, tea tree, terebinth, lemon thyme

Application methods: Bath, compress, diffuser, massage, friction/unguent

Blennorrhea

Lavender, oregano, Mysore sandalwood, red thyme

Application methods: Bath, massage, friction/unguent

Boils

Chamomile (blue, Roman, German), everlasting

Application methods: Compress, facials, mask, lotion, face oil/body oil

Bronchitis

Benzoin resinoid, lime, myrtle, niaouli, oregano, peppermint, rosemary, spearmint, spruce, tea tree, terebinth, lemon thyme
Application methods: Bath, compress, diffuser, massage

Bruises

Blue chamomile, geranium, lavender, everlasting
Application methods: Compress, lotion, friction/ unguent

Burns

Geranium, lavender, lavandin, niaouli, oregano, rosemary, spike, lemon thyme
Application methods: Compress, lotion, friction/ unguent

Candida

Tea tree
Application methods: Compress, lotion, face oil/ body oil, friction/unguent, douche

Catarrhal Condition

Frankincense, hyssop, lavender, lime, myrrh, niaouli, oregano, peppermint, rosemary, spearmint, lemon thyme
Application methods: Diffuser

Cellulitis

Angelica root, birch, cypress, fennel, geranium, grapefruit, lemon, red thyme
Application methods: Bath, compress, massage, friction/unguent, body wrap

Circulation

Cinnamon bark, cinnamon leaf, cypress, lemon, oregano, red thyme
Application methods: Bath, compress, massage, friction/unguent, body wrap

Circulation (Capillary)

Oregano, red thyme
Application methods: Bath, compress, lotion, massage, face oil/body oil, friction/unguent, body wrap

Colds

Eucalyptus globulus, lavender, pine, spruce, terebinth
Application methods: Compress, diffuser, massage, friction/unguent

Convalescence

Angelica root, carrot seed, coriander seeds, cumin seeds, lemon, lime, petitgrain biguarade
Application methods: Bath, diffuser, massage

Cough

Benzoin resinoid, cypress, frankincense, myrrh
Application methods: Diffuser

Cystitis

Birch, cajeput, cedarwood, juniper, lavender, lovage root, oregano, Mysore sandalwood, red thyme
Application methods: Bath, compress, massage, friction/unguent

Debility

Rosemary, Spanish sage, savory, lemon thyme, red thyme
Application methods: Bath, diffuser, massage

Diabetes

Eucalyptus australiana, E. globulus, geranium, juniper
Application methods: Bath, massage

Digestive Problems

Angelica root, aniseed, bergamot, Roman chamomile, German chamomile, caraway seeds, cardamom, cinnamon bark, coriander seeds, cumin seeds, fennel, gingerroot, grapefruit, lemon, lemongrass, lime, Litsea cubeba, lovage root
Application methods: Bath, compress, massage

Dyspepsia

Basil, caraway seeds, clove buds, gingerroot, hyssop, pennyroyal (use internally only with guidance of primary care practitioner), pepper, peppermint, petitgrain biguarade, spearmint, tangerine, tarragon
Application methods: Compress, massage, friction/unguent

Energy Deficiency

Caraway seeds, clove buds, cypress
Application methods: Bath, diffuser, massage

Energy Imbalance

Benzoin resinoid, cajeput, *Eucalyptus australiana, E. globulus,* myrtle, niaouli
Application methods: Bath, diffuser, massage

Fainting

Peppermint
Application methods: Compress, diffuser

Female Reproductive System

Chamomile (Roman, German), clary sage, fennel, mugwort, rose
Application methods: Bath, compress, diffuser, massage, friction/unguent, douche

Fermentations

Caraway seeds, clove buds, tarragon
Application methods: Bath, compress, massage

Fever

Gingerroot, peppermint
Application methods: Bath, compress, massage, friction/unguent

Flatulence

Cardamom, coriander seeds, cumin seeds, fennel, gingerroot, lovage root, nutmeg, petitgrain biguarade, tangerine
Application methods: Bath, compress, massage, friction/unguent

Fleas

Lavender, lavandin, pennyroyal, spike
Application methods: Diffuser, friction/unguent

Frigidity

Clary sage, jasmine absolute, rose, ylang-ylang
Application methods: Bath, compress, diffuser, massage, friction/unguent

Fungal Infections

Cedarwood, patchouli, tea tree
Application methods: Compress, lotion, friction/ unguent, douche

Gallbladder Congestion

Lemon, lime, rosemary
Application methods: Bath, compress, massage, friction/unguent

Gastric Spasms

Basil, gingerroot, tarragon
Application methods: Compress, massage, friction/unguent

Genitourinary Infections

Fir, juniper, pine, terebinth
Application methods: Bath, compress, lotion, massage

Glandular System

Carrot seed, cedarwood, coriander seeds, fennel, fir, juniper, pine, spruce, terebinth
Application methods: Bath, massage, friction/ unguent

Gout

Angelica root, coriander seeds
Application methods: Compress, massage, friction/unguent

Headache

Chamomile mixta, chamomile (Roman, German), lavender, peppermint, rosewood, spearmint
Application methods: Bath, compress, diffuser, massage, friction/unguent

Hemorrhage

Everlasting, geranium, rose
Application methods: Compress, lotion, friction/ unguent

Hemorrhoids

Cypress
Application methods: Compress, lotion, friction/ unguent

Hepatobiliary Disorders

Carrot seed, mugwort, pennyroyal, peppermint, spearmint
Application methods: Bath, compress, massage, friction/unguent

Herpes

Lemon, tea tree
Application methods: Compress, face oil/ body oil, friction/unguent

Hiccups

Tarragon
Application methods: Compress, massage, friction/unguent

Hypertension

Lemon, marjoram, ylang-ylang
Application methods: Bath, massage, friction/ unguent

Hypotension

Hyssop, Spanish sage
Application methods: Compress, diffuser, massage, friction/unguent

Immune System (Low)

Lemon, tea tree
Application methods: Bath, diffuser, massage

Impotence

Cardamom, champaca flowers, clary sage, clove buds, gingerroot, jasmine absolute, nutmeg, pepper, peppermint, rose, Mysore sandalwood, ylang-ylang
Application methods: Bath, compress, massage, friction/unguent

Infectious Diseases

Bay, cajeput, cinnamon bark, cinnamon leaf, citronella, clove buds, Eucalyptus australiana, E. citriodora, E. globulus, geranium, lavender, lavandin, lemon, lemongrass, Litsea cubeba, myrtle, niaouli, oregano, peppermint, savory, tea tree, red thyme
Application methods: Bath, compress, diffuser, massage, friction/unguent

Inflamed Joint

Chamomile (blue, German, Roman)
Application methods: Bath, compress, friction/unguent

Inflammations

Frankincense, myrrh
Application methods: Compress, facials, mask, lotion, friction/unguent

Insomnia

Chamomile mixta, chamomile (German, Roman), cistus, lavender, marjoram, wild Spanish marjoram, melissa, neroli, orange, spikenard, tangerine, lemon thyme, ylang-ylang
Application methods: Bath, diffuser, massage, friction/unguent

Insufficient Milk (Nursing)

Fennel
Application methods: Compress, massage, friction/unguent

Intestinal Infections

Basil, bergamot, cinnamon (bark, leaf), red thyme
Application methods: Compress, massage, friction/unguent

Intestines

Lovage root, nutmeg
Application methods: Bath, compress, massage

Kidneys

Birch, geranium, lovage root
Application methods: Bath, compress, massage, friction/unguent

Liver

Chamomile mixta, chamomile (blue, German, Roman), everlasting
Application methods: Compress, massage, friction/unguent

Liver and Spleen Congestion

Chamomile (German, Roman), everlasting, lemon, lemon verbena, lime
Application methods: Compress, massage, friction/unguent

Lymphatic System and Secretions

Grapefruit, lemon, lime
Application methods: Bath, massage, friction/unguent

Menopause

Chamomile mixta, chamomile (German, Roman), geranium, jasmine absolute, lavender, mugwort, Spanish sage, ylang-ylang
Application methods: Bath, compress, diffuser, massage, friction/unguent

Metabolism

Lavender, melissa, oregano, peppermint, rosemary, Spanish sage, spearmint, lemon thyme, red thyme
Application methods: Bath, diffuser, massage, friction/unguent

Migraine

Angelica root, aniseed, basil, chamomile mixta, chamomile (German, Roman), caraway seeds, coriander seeds, cumin seeds, gingerroot, lavender, marjoram, wild Spanish marjoram, melissa, peppermint, spearmint
Application methods: Compress, diffuser, friction/unguent

Mosquitos

Citronella, geranium, lavandin, pennyroyal
Application methods: Diffuser, lotion, friction/unguent

Moths

Lavender, lavandin
Application methods: Diffuser, friction/unguent

Nausea

Peppermint, rosewood, spearmint
Application methods: Compress, diffuser, massage, friction/unguent

Neuralgia

Bay, clove buds, nutmeg, pepper, peppermint
Application methods: Bath, compress, massage, friction/unguent

Obesity

Angelica root, birch, fennel, grapefruit, lemon, lime, orange, red thyme
Application methods: Bath, compress, massage, friction/unguent, body wrap

Pain (Muscular and Articular)

Bay, birch, clove buds, nutmeg, oregano, pepper, peppermint, rosemary, spike
Application methods: Bath, compress, massage, friction/unguent

Palpitations

Lavender, melissa, neroli, lemon thyme, spikenard, ylang-ylang
Application methods: Bath, compress, diffuser, massage

Perspiration (Especially Feet)

Cypress, sage
Application methods: Bath, compress, lotion, massage, friction/unguent

Premenstrual Syndrome

Carrot seed, clary sage, fennel, lavender, marjoram, mugwort
Application methods: Bath, compress, massage, friction/unguent, douche

Respiratory System

Bay, cajeput, cedarwood, clove buds, cypress, Eucalyptus australian, E. globulus, fir, hyssop, lavender, lavandin, myrtle, niaouli, oregano, peppermint, pine, rosemary, spearmint, spike, spruce, tea tree, terebinth
Application methods: Bath, compress, diffuser, massage, friction/unguent

Respiratory Weakness

Fir, pine, spruce
Application methods: Bath, diffuser, massage, friction/unguent

Rheumatism

Birch, cajeput, coriander seeds, gingerroot, juniper, marjoram, wild Spanish marjoram, nutmeg, pepper, rosemary, savory, red thyme
Application methods: Bath, compress, massage, friction/unguent

Sanitation

Citronella, *Eucalyptus citriodora,* lavandin, lemongrass, *Litsea cubeba*
Application methods: Diffuser

Secretions

Benzoin resinoid, elemi, frankincense, grapefruit, lemon, lime, myrrh
Application methods: Bath, compress, massage, friction/unguent

Sinusitis

Cajeput, *Eucalyptus australiana, E. globulus,* lavender, myrtle, niaouli, peppermint, spearmint
Application methods: Diffuser, friction/unguent

Sore Throat

Geranium, gingerroot, myrrh, pine, spruce, terebinth
Application methods: Friction/unguent, gargle

Spasms, Digestive

Angelica root, aniseed, caraway seeds, coriander seeds, cumin seeds, fennel, marjoram, wild Spanish marjoram
Application methods: Bath, compress, massage, friction/unguent

Tachycardia

Lemon verbena, spikenard, ylang-ylang
Application methods: Bath, compress, diffuser, massage, friction/unguent

Teething Pain

Chamomile (blue, German, Roman), mugwort
Application methods: Friction/unguent, gargle

Tonsillitis

Blue chamomile, geranium, gingerroot
Application methods: Friction/unguent, gargle

Toothache

Chamomile, (blue, German, Roman), clove buds, mugwort
Application methods: Friction/unguent, gargle

Tuberculosis

Cajeput, *Eucalyptus australiana, E. globulus,* myrtle, niaouli, tea tree
Application methods: Bath, compress, diffuser, massage, friction/unguent

Urinary Infections

Cajeput, cedarwood, cistus, clove buds, *Eucalyptus australiana, E. globulus,* fir, juniper, myrtle, niaouli, pine, tea tree, terebinth
Application methods: Bath, compress, massage

Varicosis

Cypress, lemon
Application methods: Compress, lotion, friction/unguent

Viral Diseases

Lemon, melissa, oregano
Application methods: Diffuser, massage, friction/unguent

Vital Centers

Basil, gingerroot, hyssop, lavender, melissa, oregano, peppermint, rosemary, Spanish sage, spearmint, lemon thyme, red thyme
Application methods: Bath, diffuser, massage, friction/unguent

Vomiting

Peppermint, spearmint
Application methods: Compress, massage, friction/unguent

Water Retention

Angelica root, birch, cypress, fennel, grapefruit, lemon, lime, lovage root, orange
Application methods: Bath, compress, massage, friction/unguent, body wrap

Whooping Cough

Cypress, hyssop
Application methods: Compress, diffuser, massage

Wounds

Benzoin resinoid, everlasting, geranium, lavender, lavandin, niaouli, oregano, rosemary, spike, lemon thyme
Application methods: Compress, lotion, friction/unguent

Wounds (Infected)

Caraway seeds, clove buds, elemi, frankincense, myrrh, tea tree
Application methods: Compress, facials, lotion, face oil/body oil, friction/unguent

MIND, EMOTIONS, AND PSYCHE

Anger
Chamomile (German, Roman), ylang-ylang
Application methods: Bath, diffuser, massage, friction/unguent

Anxiety
Benzoin resinoid, bergamot, cedarwood, fir, jasmine absolute, lemon, lime, patchouli, petitgrain biguarade, pine, rosewood, spikenard, spruce
Application methods: Bath, diffuser, massage, friction/unguent

Astral Body
Lavender, lavandin, marjoram, melissa, patchouli, rosemary, lemon thyme
Application methods: Bath, diffuser, massage, friction/unguent

Confidence (Lack of)
Jasmine absolute
Application methods: Bath, diffuser, massage, friction/unguent

Confusion
Petitgrain biguarade
Application methods: Bath, diffuser, massage, friction/unguent

Depression
Bergamot, clary sage, geranium, jasmine absolute, lavender, lemon, lime, melissa, peppermint, petitgrain biguarade, rose, rosemary, Spanish sage, Mysore sandalwood, spearmint, lemon thyme, red thyme, ylang-ylang

Application methods: Bath, diffuser, massage

Depression (Postnatal)
Clary sage, jasmine absolute
Application methods: Bath, diffuser, massage

Dream
Mugwort, clary sage
Application methods: Diffuser, friction/unguent

Emotional Shock
Melissa, neroli, rose
Application methods: Bath, diffuser, massage, friction/unguent

Fatigue (Nervous or Intellectual)
Basil, clove buds, juniper, nutmeg
Application methods: Bath, diffuser, massage

Grief
Melissa, neroli, rose
Application methods: Bath, diffuser, massage, friction/unguent

Hysteria
Neroli, orange, tangerine
Application methods: Bath, diffuser, massage

Memory (Poor)
Basil, clove buds, gingerroot, juniper, petitgrain biguarade, rosemary
Application methods: Bath, diffuser, massage, friction/unguent

Mental Fatigue, Mental Strain

Basil, caraway seeds, gingerroot, peppermint, petitgrain biguarade, rosemary, Spanish sage, spearmint

Application methods: Bath, diffuser, massage, friction/unguent

Mind

Frankincense, myrrh

Application methods: Bath, diffuser, massage, friction/unguent

Nervous System

Bergamot, cedarwood, cinnamon bark, cumin seeds, fir, lemon, lime, pepper, peppermint, petitgrain biguarade, pine, Spanish sage, savory, spearmint, spruce, lemon thyme

Application methods: Bath, diffuser, massage, friction/unguent

Nervous Tension

Geranium, lavender, marjoram, wild Spanish marjoram, melissa, neroli, orange, rose, tangerine, ylang-ylang

Application methods: Bath, diffuser, massage, friction/unguent

Nervousness

Cistus, neroli, orange, tangerine, lemon verbena

Application methods: Bath, diffuser, massage, friction/unguent

Neurasthenia

Lavender, melissa, patchouli, peppermint, rosemary, Spanish sage, spearmint, lemon thyme, red thyme

Application methods: Bath, diffuser, massage

Neurovegetative System

Basil, gingerroot, lemon verbena

Application methods: Bath, diffuser, massage, friction/unguent

Psychic Centers

Cistus, elemi, frankincense, myrrh

Application methods: Diffuser, friction/unguent

Psychic Work

Cedarwood, cistus, mugwort, spruce

Application methods: Diffuser, friction/unguent

Sadness

Benzoin resinoid, jasmine absolute, rose, rosewood

Application methods: Bath, diffuser, massage, friction/unguent

Stress

Cedarwood, fir, pine, spruce, ylang-ylang

Application methods: Bath, diffuser, massage

Tantrum

Chamomile (German, Roman)

Application methods: Bath, diffuser, massage, friction/unguent

Ungroundedness

Pepper, vetiver

Application methods: Bath, diffuser, massage, friction/unguent

Yoga, Meditation, Rituals

Cedarwood, cistus, Mysore sandalwood, spruce
Application methods: Diffuser, friction/unguent

CHAKRAS AND ENERGY CENTERS

Crown Chakra

Benzoin resinoid, cistus, frankincense, myrrh, Mysore sandalwood, spruce
Application methods: Diffuser, friction/unguent

Heart Chakra

Benzoin resinoid, melissa, neroli, rose
Application methods: Diffuser, friction/unguent

Root Chakra

Pepper, spikenard, vetiver
Application methods: Massage, friction/unguent

Sacral Chakra

Champaca flowers, jasmine absolute, ylang-ylang
Application methods: Bath, diffuser, massage, friction/unguent

Third Eye

Cistus, frankincense, myrrh, Mysore sandalwood, spruce
Application methods: Diffuser, friction/unguent

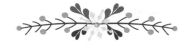

Resource Guide

Back in 1990, when this humble workbook was first published, there were only a handful of suppliers, even fewer training centers, and just a few dozen reputable retailers and treatment centers in the United States.

Today essential oils and aromatherapy products are available all across the Internet as well as from thousands of brick-and-mortar retailers. Most spas and many beauty salons offer some kind of aromatherapy treatments. Spas themselves have proliferated, and most upscale hotels now have spa facilities.

I had to limit my ambition in the actualization of this resource guide. For it to be meaningful and not arbitrary, I renounced trying to come up with a list of retailers or treatment centers, and I've reduced myself to listing only associations and the major suppliers, aware that I am leaving out lots of very good small retailers and growers. Look around wherever you live; a good many local suppliers are thriving across the country.

ASSOCIATIONS

National Association for Holistic Aromatherapy (NAHA)

naha.org

A member-based nonprofit association devoted to the holistic integration of aromatherapy into a wide range of complementary health care practices, including self-care and home pharmacy. It offers scientific, empirical, and current information about aromatherapy and essential oils to the public, practitioners, businesses, product designers, bloggers/writers, educators, health-care professionals, and media.

Alliance of International Aromatherapists (AIA)

www.alliance-aromatherapists.org

AIA is dedicated to the education of aromatherapists, health care professionals, and the public in all aspects of aromatherapy. They are a network of professionals who collectively strive to advance the profession of aromatherapy and to serve the public. Check their resources guide for publications and international associations.

International Federation of Professional Aromatherapists (IFPA)

https://ifparoma.org

The IFPA is the largest aromatherapy-specific professional practitioner organization in the United Kingdom. It works to support aromatherapists and improve standards of education and practice in aromatherapy. It is growing internationally.

EDUCATION

NAHA has an extensive listing of dozens of aromatherapy training centers at

https://naha.org/education/approved-schools

The most reputable and longest-established aromatherapy education facilities are

+ Atlantic Institute of Aromatherapy (https://atlanticinstitute.com)
+ Institute of Integrative Aromatherapy (www.aroma-rn.com)
+ Jeanne Rose's Institute of Aromatic Studies (www.jeannerose.net/courses.html)
+ Michael Scholes School of Aromatic Studies (www.michaelscholes.com)
+ New York Institute of Aromatic Studies (https://aromaticstudies.com)
+ Pacific Institute of Aromatherapy (www.pacific instituteofaromatherapy.com)
+ Tisserand Institute (https://tisserand institute.org)

PUBLICATIONS

Aromatherapy Today
an international aromatherapy journal since 1995 (www.aromatherapytoday.com)

International Journal of Clinical Aromatherapy (www.ijca.net)

International Journal of Professional Holistic Aromatherapy (www.ijpha.com)

SUPPLIERS

The aromatherapy marketplace has changed tremendously since 1990, when this workbook was first published. Back then there was a handful of reputable suppliers. There are now dozens and dozens, if not hundreds, of companies competing for the aromatherapy market, each claiming to be purer than pure. Here is a brief list of very reputable companies that have withstood the proof of time. I have deliberately avoided listing any of the numerous multilevel marketing companies, as the multilevel business model requires enormous markups from the cost of goods to the consumer price, and such high consumer prices are often justified by extravagant and even outrageous claims, with often cultish undertones. Most companies listed below offer a wide selection of essential oils of equal or much greater quality at a fraction of the cost of typical multilevel suppliers.

Eden Botanicals

edenbotanicals.com

Founded in 1985, Eden Botanicals began by importing genuine amber resin. It now carries more than 260 pure and natural essential oils, absolutes, and CO_2 extracts, including many that are rare and precious.

Frontier Cooperative Herbs (manufacturer)

www.frontiercoop.com

Frontier Cooperative Herbs is one of the largest herb distributors in the United States. Its essential oils division, Aura Cacia (www.auracacia.com), offers a wide selection of aromatherapy products. The company's products are sold primarily through health food stores.

Laboratory of Flowers

www.labofflowers.com

Founded by my friend and ex-teaching partner Michael Scholes, who has been involved in aromatherapy since 1989, the Laboratory of Flowers offers one of the largest collections of essential oils anywhere in the world, with more than six hundred essential oils from multiple species, countries of origin, and extraction methods, including more than two hundred of organic origin, along with wildcrafted oils, conventional oils, absolutes, and CO_2 extracted oils.

Mountain Rose Herbs (retailer and wholesaler)

www.mountainroseherbs.com

Grower, processor, distributor, and retailer of herbs, spices, teas, essential oils, and DIY ingredients used in herbalism. From humble beginnings in 1987 with famed herbalists Rosemary Gladstar and Rose Madrone, MRH has grown into the second-largest supplier of organic herbal products in the USA. MRH

has a strictly organic and ethical wild harvesting policy for all products. It also has implemented a zero waste and responsible packaging program. MRH is fair-trade certified by IMO's Fair for Life program.

NOW Foods

www.nowfoods.com/essential-oils

A leader in the natural products industry since 1968, NOW carries an extensive line of essential oils at reasonable prices.

Original Swiss Aromatics (manufacturer)

www.originalswissaromatics.com

Founded by Dr. Kurt Schnaubelt in 1983, Original Swiss Aromatics was one of the very first aromatherapy companies in the United States and maintains the highest standards for the more than two hundred essential oils. Original Swiss Aromatics offers a wide choice of essential oils, mostly of wild or organic origins, as well as skin and body care products. Its education division, the Pacific Institute of Aromatherapy (www.pacificinstituteofaromatherapy.com), offers a variety of courses and seminars.

Oshadhi (importer from Germany)

www.oshadhiusa.com

Oshadhi carries a comprehensive range of essential oils, many of wild or organic origins, along with skin care, body care, and fragrance products. The company's products can be found in many health food stores.

**Simplers Botanicals
(manufacturer)**

https://simplers.com

For more than thirty-two years Simplers Botanicals has been a leading source of therapeutic-quality, certified-organic essential oils and herbal extracts, with more than a hundred essential oils, therapeutic perfumes, hydrosols, infused and carrier oils, topical blends, and facial treatments.

Canada

New Directions Aromatics

www.newdirectionsaromatics.com

Established in 1997, New Directions Aromatics is a leading wholesale supplier of 100 percent pure essential oils, natural raw materials, and specialty packaging. Beginning with only a handful of distilleries, they presently source directly from ethical producers on all six continents.

Zayat Aromas

www.zayataroma.com/en

Zayat Aroma is a family enterprise committed to offering the best in holistic aromatherapy since 1985. They specialize in the distillation and distribution of pure essential oils and other aromatic products. (*Zayat* in Arabic means "the one who makes oils.") Their organic products are certified by Ecocert Canada.

Brazil

Laszlo

www.emporiolaszlo.com.br

Laszlo has the largest selection of essential oils for aromatherapy in Latin America, with more than three hundred varieties available, as well as a cosmetics line, perfumery, and more. The company functions as retailer, publisher (Editora Laszlo), and educator (Laszlo Institute) in Brazil.

United Kingdom (with International Presence)

Neal's Yard Remedies

www.nealsyardremedies.com

Established in 1981, Neal's Yard Remedies is a modern apothecary, creating award-winning natural and organic health and beauty. From small beginnings in a quiet corner of Covent Garden, they are now a global leader with a growing presence across five continents.

Tisserand Aromatherapy

www.tisserand.com

The company is named after Robert Tisserand, the author of several popular aromatherapy books and a consultant for Tisserand Aromatherapy. The company offers essential oils and skin and body care products, which can be purchased in health food stores and boutiques.

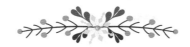

Selected Bibliography

Bardeau, Fabrice. *La Medecine par les Fleurs,* 1976.

Belaiche, P., and M. Girault, eds. *Traité de Phytotherapie et d'Aromatherapie,* vol. 3. Paris: Maloine Editeur, 1979.

Provides extensive clinical data. P. Belaiche teaches aromatherapy in French medical schools.

Cunningham, Scott. *Magical Aromatherapy.* St. Paul, MN: Llewellyn Publications, 1990.

Explores different avenues for the uses of essential oils. Comprehensive and well written.

Davis, Patricia. *Aromatherapy: An A–Z.* Saffron Walden (Essex, England): C. W. Daniel, 1988.

Patricia Davis founded the London School of Aromatherapy.

Franchomme, P., and D. Pénoël. *L'Aromathérapie exactement.* Limoges: Roger Jollois, 1990.

Gattefossé, R. M. *Aromatherapy.* Paris: Girardot, 1928.

Gattefossé coined the term *aromatherapy.*

Jackson, Judith. *Scentual Touch.* New York: Henry Holt, 1986.

Leclerc, H. *Précis de Phytotherapie.* Paris: Masson, 1954.

Maury, Marguerite. *The Secret of Life and Youth,* 1961.

Once a collector's item, now available as *Mme. Maury's Guide to Aromatherapy.* Saffron Walden (Essex, England): C. W. Daniel, 1988.

Price, Shirley. *Practical Aromatherapy.* Rochester, VT: Thorsons Publishing Group, 1983.

Ryman, Danielle. *The Aromatherapy Handbook.* Saffron Walden (Essex, England): C. W. Daniel, 1984.

Tisserand, Robert. *Aromatherapy to Heal and Tend the Body.* Wilmot, WI: Lotus Light, 1989.

Some interesting case studies.

Tisserand, Robert. *The Art of Aromatherapy.* New York: Destiny Books, 1977. The British classic.

Valnet, Jean. *The Practice of Aromatherapy.* Paris: Maloine, 1964 [American translation: Destiny Books, New York].

Still a classic, by the man who launched the revival of aromatherapy in France.

Valnet, J., C. Durrafourd, and J. C. Lapraz. *Phytotherapie et Aromatherapie: Une medecine nouvelle.* Paris: Presses de la Renaissance, 1979.

Worwood, Valerie. *Aromantics.* London: Pan Books, 1987.

Funny, well written, provocative. Certainly a different perspective.

Worwood, Valerie. *The Complete Book of Essential*

Oils and Aromatherapy. San Rafael, CA: New World Library, 1991.

Worwood, Valerie *The Fragrant Mind.* London: Doubleday, 1995.

ANTHROPOSOPHY

Goethe. *Metamorphose des plantes.* Paris: Editions Triades.

Gumbel, Dietrich. *Principles of Holistic Skin Therapy with Herbal Essences.* Heidelberg, Germany: Karl F. Haug Publishers, 1986.

Pelikan, Wilhelm. *Heilpflanzenkunde,* two volumes. Paris: Editions Triades, 1962.
Absolutely fascinating. Explains in great detail the energy aspect of medicinal plants and the botanical family approach. Available only in German and French.

ESSENTIAL OILS (PRODUCTION)

Arctander, Steffen. *Perfume and Flavor Materials of Natural Origin.* Self-published, 6665 Valley View Blvd., Las Vegas, NV 89118, 1960.

Guenther, E. *The Essential Oils,* vol. 4, 1948–1952.
Seventy years later, still the bible. For serious, committed readers only (over 10,000 pages).

Lawrence, Brian. *Essential Oils, 1976–1978, 1979–1980, 1981–1987,* three volumes. Wheaton, IL: Allured Publishing.
Reprints from Dr. Lawrence's columns in *Perfumer & Flavorist.* If Guenther is the bible, Lawrence could become the new testament. For experts only.

PERFUMERY, COSMETICS, AND FRAGRANCES

Gattefossé, R. M., and H. Jonquieres. *Technique of Beauty Products.* London: L. Hill, 1949.

Genders, Roy. *A History of Scents.* London: Hamilton, 1972.

Gibbons, Boyd. "The Intimate Sense of Smell." *National Geographic,* Sept. 1986.
Still a major landmark for the public awareness of the psychological effects of fragrances. Came with a very successful scratch and sniff test.

McKenzie, D. *Aromatics and the Soul.* London: Heinemann, 1923.

Miller, Richard and Iona. *The Magical and Ritual Use of Perfumes,* Rochester, VT: Inner Traditions, 1990.

Moncrieff, R. W. *Odours.* London: Heinemann, 1970.

Morris, Edwin T. Fragrance: *The Story of Perfume from Cleopatra to Chanel.* New York: Charles Scribner's Sons, 1984.

Poucher, William A. *Perfumes, Cosmetics and Soaps,* three volumes. Princeton: Van Nostrad, 1958.

Rimmel, E. *The Book of Perfumes.* London, 1865.

Theimer, Ernst. *Fragrance Chemistry: The Science of the Sense of Smell.* San Diego: Academic Press, 1982.

Thompson, C. J. S. *The Mystery and Lure of Perfumes.* Philadelphia: Lippincott, 1927.

Van Toller, Steve, and George Dodd, eds. *Perfumery: The Psychology and Biology of Fragrance.* London/New York: Chapman & Hall, 1988.
Conceived following the First International Conference on the Psychology of Perfumery. Fascinating. The authors conduct research at the University of Warwick in England.

TRADITION

Braunschweig, Hieronymus. *The vertuose boke of distyllacyon of the waters of all maner of herbes,* 1527.

Lemery, Nicholas. *Dictionaire des drogues simples,* 1759.

Mayer, Joseph E. *The Herbalist,* 1907.

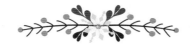

Index of Essential Oils

Bold denotes primary listings, *italics* indicate illustrations.

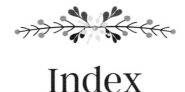

Index

Page numbers in *italics* indicate tables and illustrations.